New Life...naturally

The Home Guide to Harmonious Health

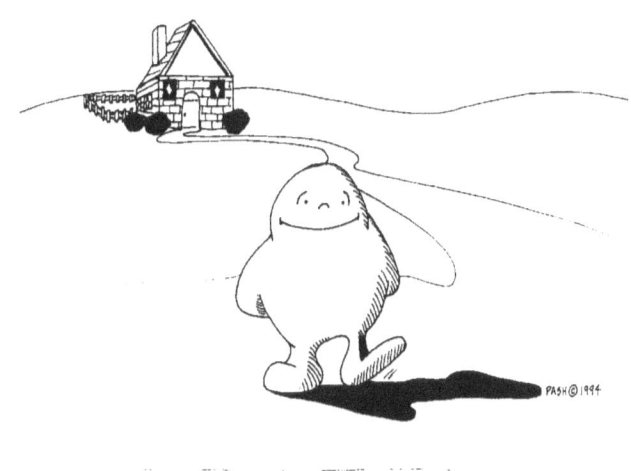

PASH © 1994

Margery Phelps

ILLUSTRATIONS
Tanya Pash & Michael Carney

FOREWORD
Janiece C. Andrews, MD

Copyright by Margery Phelps
Alpharetta, Georgia

First Published by
Croft & Sons Publishing Company
1995
Atlanta, Georgia
First Edition
ISBN 1-885857-14-4

Authored by
Margery Phelps

ISBN
13: 978-1478148814
10: 1478148810

Dedication

This book is dedicated to my Mom,

Margery Robinson Borom.

Her life taught me about beauty;

her death taught me about life.

Thousands have studied disease.
Almost no one has studied health.

- Adele Davis

AN IMPORTANT NOTICE TO THE READER:

This book is for informational and general knowledge purposes of the reader only. No guaranteed or assumptions are made to anyone with regard to any suggestions in this book. You are urged to contact your health professional if you are experiencing any health problems.

ACKNOWLEDGEMENTS:

From **Cancer & Nutrition** by Charles B. Simone, MD © 1992, $12.95. Published by Avery Publishing Group, Inc., Garden City Park, New York, (800) 548-757. Reprinted by permission.

From The **Real Vitamin & Mineral Book** by Shari Liberman and Nancy Bruning. © 1990, $9.95. Published by Avery Publishing Group, Garden City Park, New York, (800) 548-757. Reprinted by permission.

From **Self Health** by Nathaniel Lande. © 1980, by Nathaniel Lande. Reprinted by permission of Henry Holt & Co., Inc.

From **Your Health Your Choice** by Dr. Ted M Morter, Jr. © 1990, by M. Ted Morter, Jr. Reprinted by permission of Fell Publications, Inc., Hollywood, Florida.

CONTENTS

The Lord created medicines from the earth,
and a sensible man will not disparage them.

- Ecclesiastes 38: 1-2, 4

FOREWORD

JANIECE C. ANDREWS, MD

This book is a must have for the seeker of foundational facts about how magnificently our bodies are designed to self-heal and sustain health and wellness. Concepts that, until now, have been considered too complex to be interesting are presented in a completely relevant, digestible context that keeps one riveted page after page as the perfection inherent in our amazing bodies unfolds.

This author, Margery Phelps, once again displays her passion for imparting empowering truths, based on impeccable research and study, to her readers. Clearly, her investment of time and commitment translate to a work of integrity and love.

Without much effort, the reader develops an appreciation of why the narrow scope of health care information traditional in the United States has to be enlarged to embrace models of health care that have stood the test of time, although still considered to be unconventional and alternative. This includes nutrition, acupuncture, chiropractic, homeopathy, naturopathy, massage, and other energy medicine therapies.

Clearly, the burgeoning cost of health care has not translated to a more healthy population. In fact, just the opposite has occurred.

New Life...naturally is capable of becoming a classroom classic as it is readable by the very young and the very advanced in years. It is a comprehensible guidebook in every respect and can be easily taught and grasped by students who will become inspired to take personal responsibility for making healthful nutrition and lifestyle decisions and choices.

This book has the potential to promote the vision for many more natural approaches to healing as the 'dawning of a new day in American health care' emerges, and I fully and respectfully endorse *New Life ... naturally, the home guide to harmonious health.*

Remember:

My people perish for lack of knowledge.
-Hosea 4:6

Janiece C. Andrews, MD
Camp Hill, Pennsylvania
July 2012

INTRODUCTION

Welcome to Your Home

The human body is an amazing creation—a chemical processing plant that produces electrical energy to run a complex mechanical machine. In addition, it houses mental processes and emotional feelings that set it apart from and above all other life forms on the planet earth. Each of us has had a hand in our own unique creation by choosing the foods and lifestyles that directly affect and determine the kind of body we now have because every five days we form a new stomach lining, every month we renew our skin, and every three months we replace our bones.

Yet in the United States for too long we have depended on medical doctors to repair the damage we alone have caused. We eat too much, exercise too little, pollute our bodies with chemicals, and overtax our minds and emotions with stressful careers and lifestyles.

A new day is dawning in American health care and before the next sunrise we should each ask:

What am I doing to myself?

Do I put the right nutrients into this amazing creation to keep it running at peak efficiency?

Do I exercise to keep it physically fit?

Do I set aside time each day for prayer or meditation to ease the burden of stress?

Do I enjoy life?

If you can answer *yes* to these questions, chances are you have established a state of *wellness* in which you live. You may further define your state of wellness by asking these questions:

Do I feel good all the time - or do I have certain parts that hurt or cause problems?

Do I have all the energy I need - or do I frequently run out of power before I get to the end of the day?

If you are like most Americans, you probably have some minor aches and pains that you have learned to live with. You suffer from several colds a year and an occasional bout with the flu. And you probably believe that wellness can only be reached through strict dieting, obsessive exercise routines, and Spartan life styles.

In reality, being healthy is not complicated. You do not have to be either a medical doctor, or a nutritionist, nor a physiologist, or a *health nut* to properly maintain your body. For thousands of years the human race not only lived, but thrived and flourished, without the assistance of modern medical science because we lived as companions to nature. Wellness was the norm as we foraged for ourselves, eating mainly fruits and vegetables that were either fresh and raw or sun-dried.

Herbs and other natural substances were the only treatment for illness and injury, and the use of these was prescribed by the clan healer. With nothing but the natural resources provided by a beneficent Creator civilization advanced. But the growth from rudimentary, antediluvian cultures into complex societal groups created the inevitable need to produce food to feed the masses of people who gathered in cities. There was no longer any need to forage to provide food for oneself, and this formerly inborn skill became obsolete.

A race of larger statute, greater vigor, increased longevity and higher degree of cultural attainment is the reward to the nation that uses scientific discoveries in nutrition intelligently.
- Dr. Brown, speaking at
Malvern Collegiate.[1]

Industrialization created even more separation from nature. Mass production of foodstuffs with refining processes that removed the natural and essential nutrients became the norm.

Pharmaceutical establishments began to produce synthetic vitamins to replace the misguidedly extracted natural nutrients and also brought us man-made medicines that treated only the symptoms of illness. These, too, eventually became the norm, replacing remedies of the natural healers—the people who for millions of years treated illness with herbs.

Deviations from what was natural and good for us brought new diseases as our bodies struggled to accommodate unnatural substances. This internal pollution with foreign substances induced the production of lethal free radicals and the beginning of our descent into disease. Refined sugar, defined by the natural healers as *poison*, caused diabetes, depression, and mental illness. Alcohol gave us liver diseases, and nicotine gave us lung cancer. After thousands of years of wellness, we were sick.

Economics played a hand as well. We were lead to depend more and more on drugs which produced huge incomes for their manufacturers. In the early 1900s a man by the name of Abraham Flexner was employed by the Carnegie Foundation to visit every one of the 155 medical training schools in the country to determine which ones should receive the foundation's vital funding. At that time there was little regulation over medical education, and many of the schools seemed to be economic enterprises themselves, with little or no laboratory or clinical training, and low criteria for admission.[2]

Although the idea for medical education reform may have seemed noble, Flexner himself wrote in his autobiography that 120 of these schools were forced to close.[3] Because some of the giant companies that backed these charitable foundations were some of the same companies that produced drugs, you can only wonder if their charitable endeavors had an economic basis.

Funding was withdrawn from schools that did not comply with the new criteria for students and curriculum. At that time there were only eight black medical schools in the country. Six of them were forced to close.

Every medical school that had women students also shut down.[4] In their book *Fit for Life II: Living Health*, Harvey and Marilyn Diamond say that the schools that taught natural remedies and nutrition were also opposed by Flexner and they, too, succumbed to these pressures.[5]

As the *drug lords* set standards and decided who would be admitted and what courses schools would teach, freedom of choice for health care in America died. And medical doctors (educated at schools endorsed and funded by the drug pushers) with minimal education in nutrition, and no schooling on herbs or natural remedies, took over the care of the ill and injured, using the manufactured drugs.

(You may be interested to know that the word *drug* is the opposite of the word *revive*. If you were sick, would you prefer to be drugged or revived?)

We have forgotten that health is a birthright and that illness is a manifestation of the body's attempt to repair itself. We have lost touch with the good and natural remedies that actually assist the body in its repair efforts.

Sixty percent of cancer in women and 40% in men is related to diet. Heart disease and diabetes are also the result of our dietary choices.

We have become more and more dependent upon a myriad of man-made synthetic chemicals produced by the pharmaceutical giants, and ignore the statistics that show 5 million Americans are hospitalized each year for treatment of side effects suffered from the use of these drugs. In a five-year period, poison control centers had 670,000[6] reports of children having reactions to over-the-counter drugs. In the summer of 1994 the *Journal of the American Medical Association* reported "the nation's biggest drug problem: the poor prescribing practices of doctors."[7] And, one in four elderly patients becomes ill from prescribed drugs.[8]

If we have documented proof that prescribed drugs are such a problem, why has nothing been done? Each year more than a million people are hospitalized with Adverse Drug Reactions (ADRs) and 100,000 die.

Surveys have repeatedly shown that vitamins and minerals are a prudent course of treatment and one report concluded that vitamins are 1,200 times safer than drugs approved by the FDA.

In spite of vast strides in medical science, each year we lose more and more people to cancer, diabetes, heart disease, and the most recent development in our downward spiral into illness, AIDS.

Forty percent of cancer patients die from malnutrition, and not from the cancer itself.

"There are an estimated 100,000 or more hospital deaths each year attributed to sepsis,"[9] a blood-stream infection.

If all this was not bad enough, we add to the problem by overeating—since one in three Americans is overweight.[10]   Obesity   itself   causes   many   health problems.

I am not a health professional—I had to learn these things for myself, doing independent reading and research. As journalism major in college, I always loved investigation and writing, but it never occurred to me that I would someday join the wellness crusade. Growing up in a household where topics of health were frequently discussed at the dinner table, I took my fortunate good health for granted.

My mother was a scientific and medical illustrator for the Centers for Disease Control in Atlanta, and as children my twin sister Mary and I were participants in health training films produced at CDC. Mother's drawing board at home was always cluttered with medical drawings or statistical data to be used in publications about health. And, because mother was so involved in health, she feed us a healthy diet—fresh fruits, vegetables and whole grain breads.

When I became critically ill in 1981, I was admitted to the hospital for diagnostic tests. The tests themselves were almost fatal due to the chemicals that were injected into my spine. Writhing in intractable pain, with my body contorted in a fetal position, I wondered if I would live to see my daughter and son grow to adulthood. She was fourteen and he was nine. Twelve days and many thousands of dollars later, saved only by the prayers of faithful family and friends, I was released from the hospital.

You can live to be 150 years old if you eat right.
- Dr. Flora Rose[11]

Although I survived, complete recovery took a year, and my body chemistry was permanently altered. I could not tolerate any substance that was not natural. As a result, my family's lifestyle was dramatically changed. No longer were processed foods allowed. No food coloring. No preservatives. We had to eliminate everything that was not natural to our bodies.

I found that I was on an exciting path of discovery. I wanted to understand myself—not only physically, but mentally and spiritually as well. I wanted to be well and whole again. And I wanted my children to avoid the experience that almost killed me.

In 1990, my eighty-two year old mother died from massive hemorrhages caused by medicine prescribed for asthma. Coupled with my own experience, I began to wonder what we are doing to our bodies—the precious and marvelous creations that the Lord gave each of us. Her death was tragic, and even more compelling because she had spent her life trying to make us healthy. The work she created at CDC was literally sent around the world in the name of health.

After Mom's death I started collecting news stories on health issues and drugs and subscribed to several wellness newsletters. I learned there are many nutriceutical companies manufacturing all-natural herbal, vitamin and mineral formulations that have wonderfully therapeutic benefits without the side effects of drugs. One particular formulation really struck home because it treats asthma and allergies. Of course, the nutriceutical company cannot make this claim since the policies and politics of the FDA prevent honest labeling of natural products!

The more I read the more outraged I became at what we are doing to ourselves, and how we have been blinded by the selfish economic goals of pharmaceutical companies. An article in a 1991 edition of *U.S. News & World Report* discussed the health care crisis in America and gave ten recommendations for fixing it. There was not one mention of wellness, or prevention, or natural therapies. It's been more than twenty years since that article was written and not much has improved.

Reading more and more stories such as my mother's, I was compelled to join the wellness crusade. Unlike others who honor only the natural therapies, however, I vowed not to alienate the allopathic (medical doctors) community. Not only are four of my Godchildren the offspring of doctors, but doctors wield a great deal of influence over millions of patients. And they have this power because we have failed to educate ourselves about our own bodies. But if we understand how the body functions, we can take an active role in its care.

Only by opening the eyes of the American public, and the American physicians, and showing them the many natural routes we can take to restore health, can we hope to control the mammoth toll that poor health is taking on our homeland. We much teach everyone that degenerative and immune deficiency diseases need to be addressed as a nutritional challenge first. As my former colleague Bill Downs of InterHealth says, "there is no such thing as a pharmaceutical drug that can cure a nutritional deficiency."

My extensive reading on health issues and nutrition lead naturally to a profound curiosity about the functioning of the body. What keeps this remarkable machine working? It's not just the brain, or the heart, or even the digestive system or endocrine glands. If you really want to understand the human body, it seemed to me you had to start at the cellular level.

As I abandoned a 17-year career in building and home construction to enter the most exciting career I could possibly imagine, it occurred to me that our bodies are really our homes. We invite people into our homes and they come in the front door.

The mouth is like the front door—what do you invite into your precious home?

The stomach is like the kitchen where food is prepared.

The intestinal tract and colon are the trash compactor and garbage disposal.

The brain and nervous system are the telephone, and the metabolism is the furnace.

There seemed to be many similarities between the houses I built as a contractor and the real home in which I lived as a human being. The good Lord has blessed us with these wonderful earth suits—and they are our home while we are here on planet earth.

We are really extremely complex and magnificent creations and that may be one reason more of us don't take time to find out about ourselves. It's kind of mind boggling to really understand what is going on in the body. We just do what is easy and what we have come to know, passed down to us through our heritage.

Of course, that is totally different from the original human heritage of nutrition which was virtually raw fruits and vegetables. We simply were not designed to ingest the unnatural chemicals that comprise a large part of our diets today.

What we call diseases and illnesses are merely symptoms that the entire body is out of kilter.
                                    - William Dufty[12]

I started this book with a mission: *Make health education fun by writing to Inform, Inspire and Entertain!*

My first goal is to teach people to understand their bodies so they won't suffer the way I have. When you understand how your body works, you can move out of the *fix it when it's broke* mentality and into the mode of taking responsibility for your own well being.

We need a new paradigm in health. Prevention begins with consciousness; it begins with the knowledge that the mind and the body can and do heal themselves through natural means.
                        - Robert D. Willix, Jr., M.D., FACSM

Your body is the most important home you will ever have. It is the home of a beautiful, unique person—YOU. The purpose of this book is to tell you some things about your body so you will want to take responsibility for your own well being. Through rational understanding of balanced nutrition and learning how to listen to your body to achieve metabolic and physiological harmony, you can put yourself on the road to wellness.

And if you do have a serious health challenge, you will be better equipped to discuss natural and complementary therapies with your health practitioner. To secure the wellness which is your birthright, you should have access to the essential information that will allow you to participate in the decisions regarding your body—the home in which you live.

Welcome to your Home!

CHAPTER 1

The Foundation of Your Home

Your home has many parts: Bones, muscles, cartilage, nerves, skin, hair, teeth, fingernails and toe nails, blood veins and arteries, and an assortment of organs including the brain, intestinal tract, kidneys, eyes, ears, and heart. The foundation for these parts is the cell—the basic building block of the body. And there are more than 75 trillion of them in the average human adult!

Why is it necessary to understand the cell? Because, as human beings, we live and die cell by cell. Unless you understand the basic functions of the 75 trillion cells that form your body, you probably don't appreciate the significance of proper nutrition at the cellular level. And if you don't maintain wellness at the cellular level you "may be laying the foundation for disease."[13]

Just as a house will not stand for long without a firm foundation, we are healthy only to the degree that we maintain our cells. If we are not healthy it is because we have failed to provide the necessary nutrients to our cells—our building blocks.

Perhaps if you think of each of your cells as a complete and vital person you can better understand the importance of this concept. Each cell, like an individual, must eat, process food, eliminate waste, and do some sort of specific job. To keep our society running we have a variety of trades: teachers, accountants, artists, pharmacists, nurses, musicians, beauticians, carpenters, electricians, florist, doctors, lawyers, dieticians, and on and on. Each one of these jobs is important to the overall health of our society. None is more important than the other. It takes everyone working together to provide the needs and wants of us all.

The cells in your body have specific roles, too, and to perform properly they must be supplied with the proper tools. You could not expect a carpenter to build a house with a computer any more than a concert pianist could perform Mozart on a hammer. The proper tools for your cells come from good nutrition.

This is Harmony, the Healthy Cell. We will be using Harmony throughout this book to illustrate the good and bad nutritional habits that create the condition of your home.

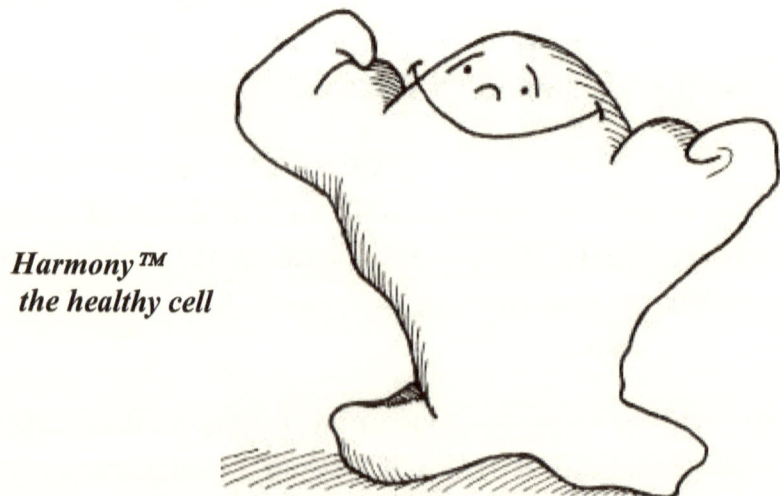

Harmony ™
the healthy cell

HOME
INSURANCE
POLICY:[14]

> *By understanding how the systems of the body work together, you will be in a better position to build a firm foundation of good health.*
> - Dr. M. Ted Morter, Jr.

In addition to eating and working habits, your individual cells have other similarities to the body as a whole: skin, support structure (skeletal system), brain, circulation, reproduction, and energy generators. Let's take a look at a few of them.

Harmony's *skin* is a membrane that encloses the cell's body. Working like an organ, the cell membrane takes food into the cell. Inside Harmony, the most predominant components are protein and water. The cell membrane is made of protein, as well as the microfilaments that line the membrane and give Harmony structural support—like your skeletal system. These supports are called the cortex or ectoplasm.

Like your body, Harmony has many organs (organelles) that perform various functions. The *brain* of the cell is the nucleus and it controls all of Harmony's activity. The nucleus also houses the DNA molecules and genes that decide what characteristics you will inherit.

The endoplasmic reticulum is a network of channels that run from Harmony's outer membrane to the double wall membrane that surrounds the nucleus. These channels serve as the transportation route for all the substances moving throughout Harmony.

Other important organs are the mitochondria. These are the cell's furnaces, where it burns fuel to provide Harmony with energy. If the cell is located in an organ that requires a lot of energy, like the heart, it will have thousands of mitochondria. But if it is located in a low-energy organ such as the eye, there may be less than a hundred.

Red blood cells are the only cells that do not have mitochondria. They are in the delivery business for the body and their major customer is the lungs. With its 25 trillion cells, the blood picks up oxygen in the lungs and hauls it to the other 50 trillion cells in your body. Red blood cells only live about 120 days but your supply is constantly replenished by their manufacturing plant, the bone marrow.

Harmony is protected by an army of white blood cells, also known as leukocytes. There are six types of leukocytes to defend Harmony from invaders such as viruses and bacteria. Needless to say, they have a short but useful life span.

By a process called mitosis Harmony can reproduce, creating an exact duplicate in ten to thirty hours. For some cells, like skin, this is a continual process. Others, like muscle, reproduce infrequently, and some never, such as teeth.

Harmony is mostly fluid—and so is your body. The fluid substance in your cells is called cytosol. It is composed of cholesterol, electrolytes, esterified fatty acids, glucose, and proteins, as well as enzymes and waste products— urea and uric acid. Enzymes (complex proteins) are the catalyst for various functions in the cell. Without proper enzymes, work won't get done.

Harmony gets food three ways: it seeps in through the membrane (diffusion), it is pushed in by other substances, or Harmony encircles it and draws it in (endocytosis). Whatever method Harmony uses, nutrients are taken from the fluid outside the cell to the fluid inside.

Supervision of Harmony comes from two sources. The nucleus has over-all control of internal operations of the cell but the body's hypothalamus is Commander-in-Chief. The hypothalamus, located in the brain, governs all life support functions—breathing, heart rate, digestive processes, blood pressure, etc.—through messages delivered by hormones that are carried through the blood to the cells.

When your cells are healthy, and free of toxins, the tissues they form will be healthy, too. When your tissues are hale and hearty, the organs they form will be strong and sound. With well maintained organs, all the systems in your home will operate at peak efficiency, and you can live in a state of wellness. But it all starts with Harmony. Because each of your cells is continuously bathed in the nutrients from which it must receive its food, and the tools it requires to perform its work, you can understand why proper nutrition is essential to good health. If the cell does not receive the proper nutrition, Harmony will die.

HOME
INSURANCE
POLICY:

> *Your home was built for Harmony, Health and Happiness.*

CHAPTER 2

The Front Door

Are you selective about the guests you invite into your home?

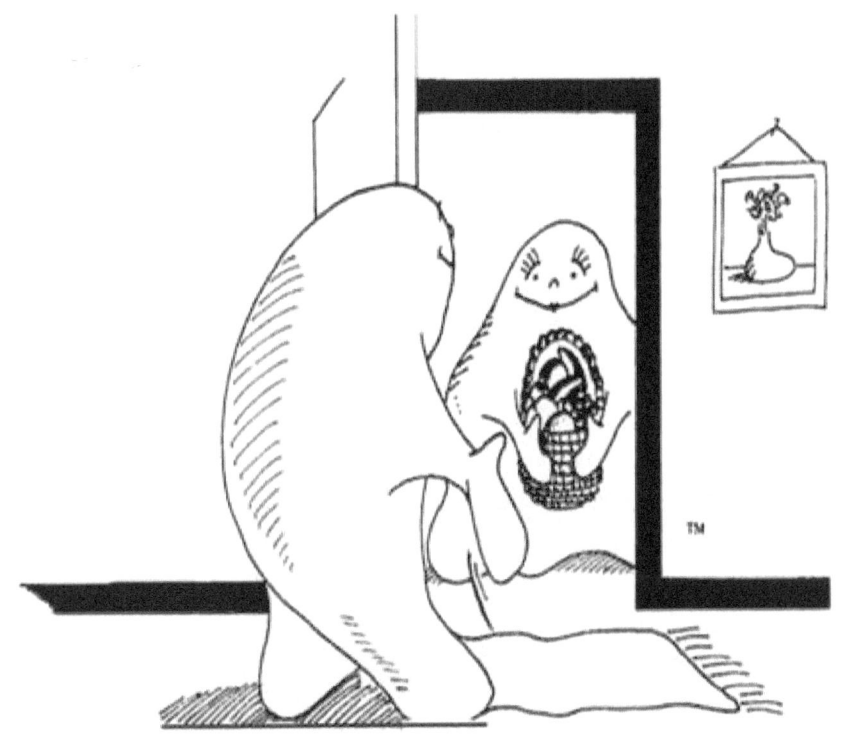

What kind of guests to you invite into your home?

We all enjoy the house guests who make their own beds, wipe the ring out of the bathtub, and wash their dirty dishes. But you don't welcome visitors if you know they will spill food, damage furniture, or stop up the toilet.

How about the food you put into your mouth?

Have you ever thought about the real effect it has on your cells?

Do you eat for nutritional health or do you eat strictly for pleasurable tastes?

Does the food you eat create chaos in your body or does it enhance your well-being?

What does your diet do to Harmony?

If you eat the typical American diet high in processed food, you are bombarding your cells with chemicals they were never designed to handle—like nitrates, nitrites, sulfates and sulfites, disodium inosinate, disodium guanylate, sodium aluminum phosphate, monosodium glutamate, and many, many others. Then, to add to this insult, we starve these precious cells of the vital nutrition they do require to maintain themselves.

HOME
INSURANCE
POLICY:[15]

You can make yourself well or ill according to the food you consume, and millions of people are unconsciously committing suicide daily at their own tables.   - Dr. Laura Newman

Deprived of essential nourishment (and different cell groups have different needs), cells weaken and start to break down. They become prime targets for illness. In essence, we give them a double whammy! We assault them and we starve them.

Is it any wonder that disease is so widespread?

Any reasonable discussion of diet must take geographic and social heritage into consideration. For example, Eskimos consume large quantities of meat, which is to be expected since their access to fresh vegetables and fruits is gravely limited. Although the prominent fat content of their diet helps provide warmth, it also contributes to a high rate of heart disease.

Orientals historically eat large quantities of rice. Generally, they do not have the obesity problems suffered by Westerners; nor do they have the related cardio-vascular diseases. There any many instances where the geographic distribution of disease indicates an important connection between nutritional habits and illness.

In the United States the rate of cancer has increased along with our increased consumption of fat, animal protein and sugar. During the past fifty years we have eaten less fiber.[16] In Finland, where a large percentage of fat comes from diary product consumption, the rate of heart attacks is high.[17] Colon cancer rates are high in Western European and the English-speaking countries[18] and low in Asia and Africa. Statistical surveys continue to provide overwhelming evidence that our health is determined by our food.

Food plays an active part in our social lives as well. Dinner parties with friends, power lunches with business associates, and holiday festivities with family all seem to create a certain degree of over-indulgence at the table.

Terribly out of balance after the feast, Harmony lets us know that we have over-stuffed our stomachs. Of course, with its innate ability to bring itself back into balance, and with proper nutrition, your body recovers from this occasional gluttony.

HOME
INSURANCE
POLICY:

> *Why is it that we punish our bodies with too much fat, too much sugar, too many rich foods, and too much alcohol when we are celebrating the special times in our lives?*

What is proper nutrition?

What do you really need to eat to make Harmony happy?

What is the best food to bring into your home?

And, how should it be prepared?

The Wall Street advertisers, thousands of processed food manufacturers, and high society food magazines have helped us forget that eating should be a normal and natural process. So, here are a few basic rules to remember:

First, if it is not natural, it is not good. Your body was designed to live on the earth and eat the foods supplied in nature. Anything else is unnatural to your Harmony. (Have you ever noticed that wild animals don't suffer from heart disease or cancer? Nor do the fishes in the sea, or the birds in the sky. Could it be because they consume only what nature provides for them?)

Second, natural means just that. Cooking, seasonings and mixing natural foods can turn it into fake food.

Third, you are what you eat!

So, what is *natural?* And what is *processed?*

Why are natural foods good guests in our homes and why does processed food make chaos out of Harmony?

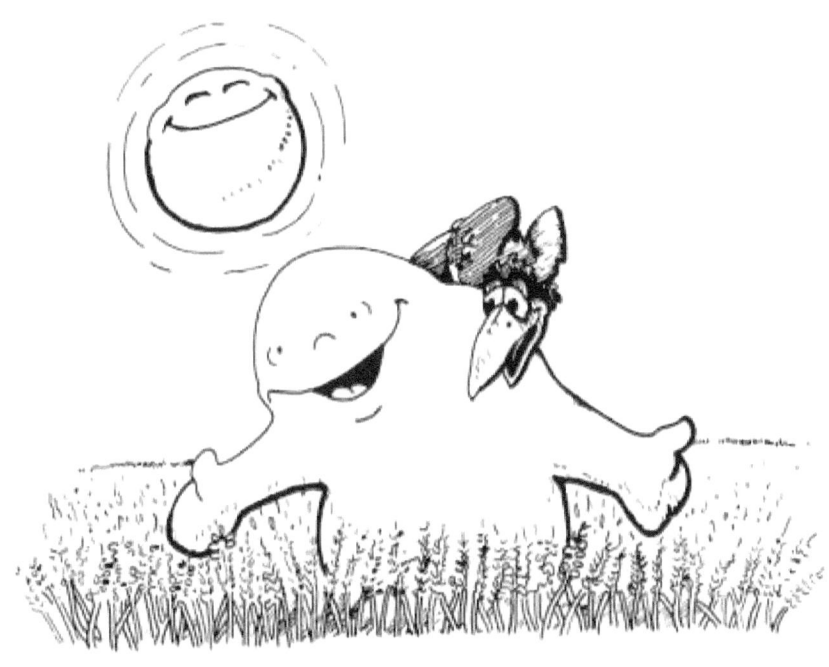

Natural food is genuine, real food. It is organic, which means it is alive. Food that has been processed or produced artificially is not alive. It is dead. Your cells are alive. Therefore, if you want them to do their work, you must provide them with live food. Dead food cannot provide the *tools* your cells need.

(Genetically Modified Food—GMO—is an entirely different discussion which I will address in my blog and another book.)

HOME
INSURANCE
POLICY:

> *I have given you every plant yielding seed that is on the surface of all the earth, and every tree which has fruit yielding seed; it shall be food for you.*   - Genesis 1:29

Take a look at a loaf of white bread. The first listed ingredient is flour. No matter what kind of flour was used, it is dead. The process to turn wheat into white flour starts with the milling, where the *living* part of the wheat is removed by grinding and refining. After numerous other procedures, including bleaching, the live, nutrient rich kernel has been turned into a fine powder. And the life has literally been beaten out of it.

Flour used for white bread has at least twenty nutrients removed through processing, including large portions of vitamin C, vitamin B-6, and zinc. Then the dutiful manufacturers replace these with a paltry portion of nutrients and put the label *enriched* on the wrapper.

This is not to say that white bread is totally void of nutrition. You do get carbohydrates and fat, and Harmony needs both. But along with them you are littering your home with numerous other chemicals and *dead* substances. They are like foreign invaders in your beautiful home.

When enough of these bad guys invade Harmony's territory, and cut off essential supply and elimination routes, Harmony has no choice except to surrender.

HOME
INSURANCE
POLICY:

Since you are what you eat, do you really want to eat dead food?

If you want to be healthy, and keep Harmony in your home, your diet should include a variety of whole grains and starches as well as legumes, fresh fruits and vegetables.

The best way to eat fruits and vegetables is raw. Fruit provides Harmony with all the essential tools: vitamins, minerals, carbohydrates for glucose and energy, calcium, phosphorus, and amino acids.

Harmony uses amino acids to build protein—a major component of the cell. Since we can only metabolize (create in our bodies) some of the twenty amino acids we require, it is vital that we get the others in our food. That's why they are called *essential* amino acids. If we don't eat them, our cells won't have them to repair and rebuild Harmony.

If your vegetables must be cooked, steam them for a few minutes. Overcooking destroys vitamins and enzymes. Vegetables also provide calcium and protein. Although we don't think of veggies as a source of protein, they are. All living matter is composed of protein so vegetables contain a good supply.

Unfortunately, many of us believe we need the dietary proteins found in meats, fish and poultry. As a result, we don't eat enough fresh vegetables. Our belief in animal source protein was first derived from research done on rats in 1914 that was promulgated by various food trade organizations, such as the National Egg Board and the Dairy Council. The researchers failed to acknowledge, and the trade associations chose to ignore, the fact that humans and rats have different nutritional requirements. Vegetables contain all the protein-producing amino acids that Harmony must have to function properly. Vegetables are also low in fat—an extra bonus—and provide fiber.

Vegetables are also an excellent source of iron. In his book *Diet for a New America*, John Robbins says, "Cow's milk is so low in iron that you'd have to drink 50 gallons to get the iron available from a single bowl of spinach."[19]

HOME
INSURANCE
POLICY:[20]

| *Healthy, properly functioning cells work in harmony with all the organs and systems...* |
| - Dr. M. Ted Morter, Jr. |

We know that disease is not the cause of poor health. Just the opposite—our eating and poor health habits are the cause of disease. Our bodies were designed to function perfectly when provided the proper nutrients— those found naturally in nature. When we cease to provide proper nutrition, we invite disease into the precious cells that make our bodies.

What do you invite into your home—Harmony or havoc?

CHAPTER 3

The Washroom

Next to air, water is the most essential element of life—your body is sixty-five to seventy-five percent water!! So if you want to keep Harmony in a state of wellness, it is vital that you bathe your cells with ample quantities of pure water. Let's take a trip to the washroom in our home and visit Harmony.

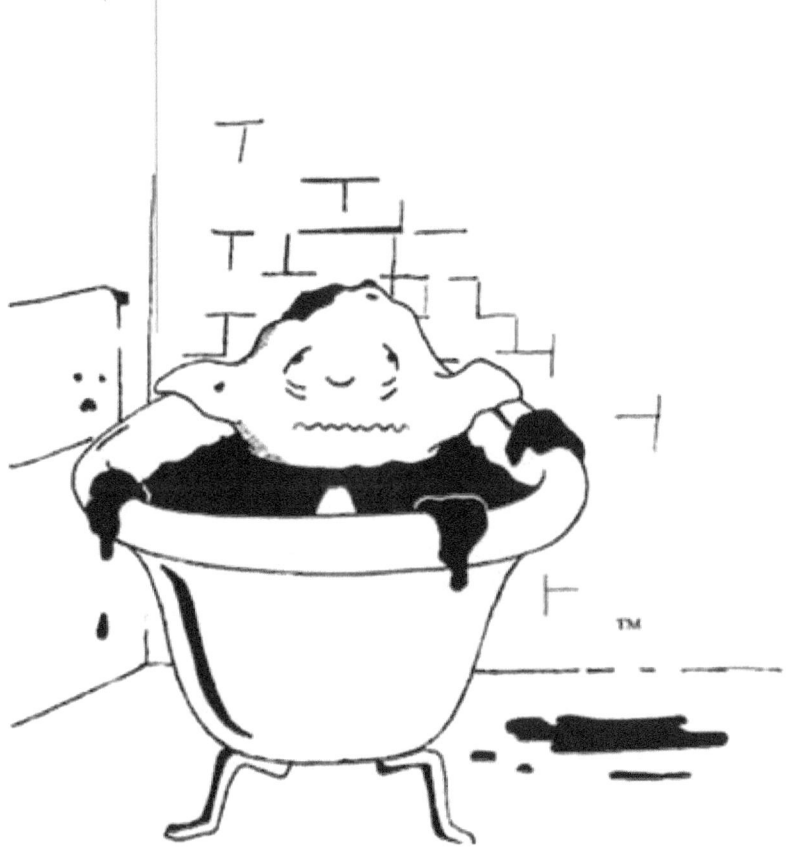

As you can see, Harmony is not too happy. Because the body did not receive enough clean water, Harmony is bathing in a bathtub full of polluted water and all those precious cells are soaking in a sea of toxins. Ugh!!

This dreadful situation might cause you to ask these questions:

- Why do you need water?

- What kind of water should you drink?

- How much water should you drink?

To answer our first question, the body requires water for every function it performs. Harmony is helpless without this huge partner in life.

Water works as a lubricant and hydrates the skin while also serving as a shock absorber to the joints, muscles and bones. Think about the bones in your feet, knees and hips.

How would they feel if you started jumping up and down and there was no cushion between them?

Your internal organs float in an ocean of nutrition that must be constantly restocked since you lose about a gallon of water a day just through the normal functions like breathing, digestion and elimination.

Just imagine how all those precious internal organs would feel if they were constantly banging against each other without the lubrication that water provides!

HOME
INSURANCE
POLICY:[21]

> *Drinks loaded with dissolved sugars or milk increase water needs, instead of satisfying them.* - Linda Rector-Page, N.D., Ph.D.

You need water for all the digestive processes. Water is essential to the production of saliva in the mouth. Can you pretend that you are putting food in your mouth and you don't have any moisture there? How could you chew your food or swallow it without saliva? In the stomach water is a vital component of the digestive juices.

Water is the major component of the body's transportation system—the blood and lymph. It picks up nutrients in the digestive tract and delivers it to the cells. When it reaches the cells, water swaps the nutrients for the toxins the cell has stored and it carries these toxins to the body's elimination systems. Without water, the nutrients don't get into Harmony and the toxins don't get out.

HOME
INSURANCE
POLICY:

> *Your body is a toxic chemical manufacturing plant that produces things like ammonia, carbon dioxide, nitrogen, and urea. These toxics must be gathered like foreign spies and exported from the body. You need water to carry them to their final elimination destination.*

Water is also needed to regulate your body's temperature. If you get over-heated, your body sweats to cool itself down. This process uses a great deal of water. If the water is not replaced, the body will become dehydrated. Over-heating and dehydration can kill you.

The kind of water you drink is the second thing for you to think about if you want to maintain Harmony and balance in the washroom. Because we are accustomed to turning on the kitchen faucet and taking a drink we don't usually stop to think about our water supply.

Do you know what's in the water you drink?

If you live in a metropolitan area anywhere in the United States chances are your water has been chlorinated and fluoridated.

Do you know what fluorine and chlorine do to the water?

Do you know what these chemicals do to your Harmony?

Since city water is known to have up to 500 kinds of bacteria, viruses and parasites, chlorine is added to many public water supplies to kill these germs.[22] Your body contains bacteria, too, and many, many of these bacteria are your friends, not foes. They are essential to proper digestion and assimilation of food in the intestinal tract.

Do you know what the chlorine in water does to these good guys?

It kills them, too, since it doesn't know the difference between the friendly bacteria and the naughty germs. In addition, chlorine is a known carcinogen. Chemical compounds created by chlorinated water have been associated with increased risk for gastrointestinal cancers. That's not a surprising statistic, is it? There was a reason for those friendly bacteria in the intestinal tract. Do you think killing them off with chlorine made the intestines an attractive home for the cancer?

HOME INSURANCE POLICY:[23]	*...a study involving 3,000 people from the U.S. National Cancer Institute suggests that chlorine may double the risk for developing urinary bladder cancer.* 　　- Dr. Charles B. Simone

Did you know that sodium fluoride, another additive to many public water supplies, is a poison?

Although some research may show fluoride has a potential benefit by reducing tooth decay, do you really want to drink a substance that is used to kill rats and cockroaches?[24] A safer and healthier way to reduce tooth decay is to reduce sugar consumption. (We'll talk more about sugar in Chapter 11.)

After throwing Harmony out of balance by bathing your cells in the carcinogens of chlorine and the poison of fluoride, American tap water takes many other contaminants into the washroom. Both copper and lead water pipes can also pose threats to your health. By leaching into your water, lead can cause brain damage and copper can upset the zinc-copper ratio in your body.[25]

HOME
INSURANCE
POLICY:[26]

> *The EPA says that drinking polluted water is one of the top four health hazards to Americans.*

In addition, the following also raise the risks that Harmony will eventually be drowned by pollution:

- Chemicals from manufacturing plants are accidentally spilled or intentionally dumped into rivers and streams that supply our water;

- Fertilizers used on lawns, gardens, and farms wash into nearby water reservoirs;

- Radioactive materials from industrial facilities, hospitals, and nuclear power plants are not properly stored and leak into the ground water; and

- Millions and millions of pounds of household garbage and refuse are dumped into landfills across the country. As it decomposes, it leaches into the underlying water table, causing contamination of untold toxicity.

With all this exposure to toxins, why would anyone drink the average American tap water?

Since your body was not designed to process the deadly chemicals found in our drinking water it is essential that contaminants be removed before consumption.

Do you want to know how you provide Harmony with good, clean water?

1. Drink distilled water, which is pure H_2O, or

2. Use a water filter certified by the Water Quality Association.

Now that you know why you need water, and what kind to drink, do you know how much you need?

According to Dr. F. Batmanghelidj, who has done extensive research on the effects of dehydration due to inadequate water consumption, "Your body needs an *absolute minimum* of six to eight 8-ounce glasses of water a day." [27]

He goes on to say that beverages such as alcohol, coffee, colas and tea, "don't count as water." [28] These drinks do contain some water, but also contain ingredients that dehydrate the body.[29]

To comfortably consume adequate amounts of water, you may want to follow Dr. Batmanghelidj's suggestion to drink one glass of water prior to meals, and another glass two and a half hours after eating. In his landmark book, *Your Body's Many Cries for Water*, Dr. Batmanghelidj describes many ailments that can be caused by dehydration of the cell.

Your activity level also affects your water requirements. If you are running a marathon or playing a vigorous game of tennis one day you will certainly need more water than the day you sit in an air conditioned office.

HOME
INSURANCE
POLICY:

> *Each body has its own individual need for water, and each body's need for water can change daily.*

Water is essential. Your life depends on it! If you want to be healthy, be sure you bring plenty of pure water to the washroom for Harmony.

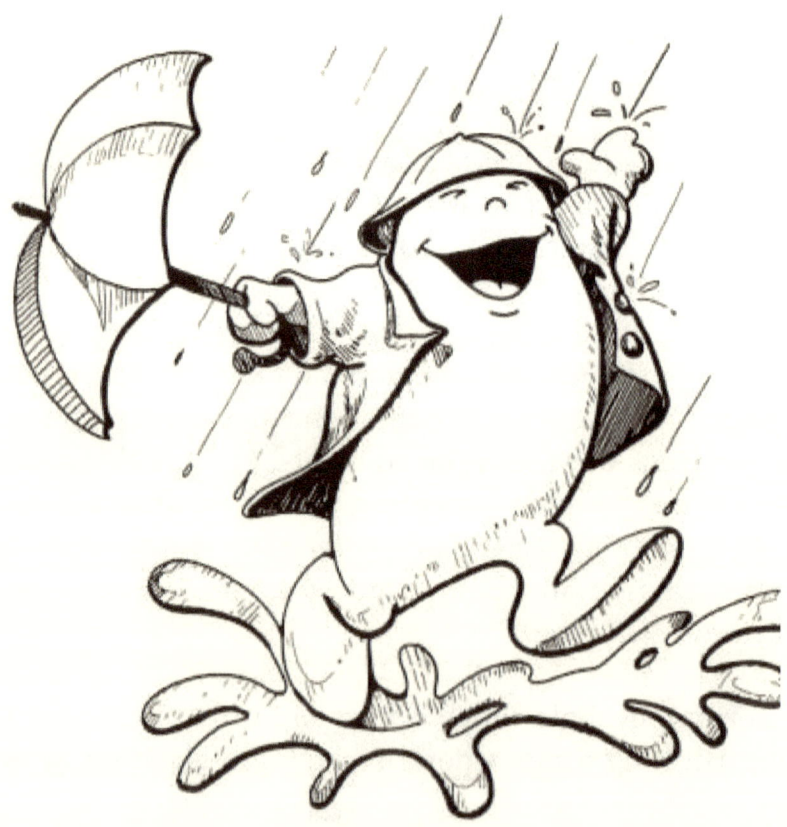

CHAPTER 4

The Kitchen - Stove, Trash Compactor and Garbage Disposal

If the mouth is the front door to your body, the digestive system would be the kitchen—the place where food is prepared for use by the cells. And just like the kitchen in your house, this process not only creates useable food for energy, but waste, which must be eliminated after all the nutritional elements have been extracted.

If the body does not eliminate waste, it builds up and you become toxic.

"The more toxic you are, the sicker you can become."[30]

If you have ever been to your county landfill and smelled the air around the piles of garbage, you can appreciate the toxicity that accumulates in the tissues and cells of your body when it is not removed.

To understand how these toxins form in the body, let's take a trip to the kitchen and see how food is prepared for your cells.

<table>
<tr><td>HOME
INSURANCE
POLICY:</td><td>When there are too many toxins in your home, Harmony will do anything to get rid of them. The name for this kind of house cleaning is "disease."</td></tr>
</table>

The process begins in the mouth, where saliva and enzymes, assisted by grinding teeth, start preparing food for your cells by breaking it down into smaller and smaller pieces. When this food reaches the stomach very acidic gastric juices, including hydrochloric acid, are used to digest the food further, breaking it down into molecules.

Now this somewhat prepared food (chyme— pronounced "kime") travels through the pyloric valve into the duodenum where glands spew mucus onto it before it enters the small intestine. This mucus keeps the very strong acid from burning the intestines. The *cooking* process continues with the addition of bile and pancreatic fluid—about two quarts a day!

Bile is produced in the liver and stored temporarily in the gall bladder. Bile must be alkaline. If it is too acidic, the bile can't neutralize the acidic chyme and the duodenum can literally be burned. This results in a duodenal ulcer and three-fourths of all ulcers are formed here.[31]

The food you eat directly affects the acids and alkaloids in your body. Fruits and vegetables generally create alkaline supplies for Harmony, but meats, grains, and dairy products add to the acid stock. Harmony was created to work in a slightly alkaline atmosphere, so too much acid can throw your body out of balance and into chaos. To get itself back into balance, the cells will take whatever mineral reserves they need from somewhere else in the body. Alkaline minerals include calcium, magnesium, potassium, and sodium.

Since calcium is necessary for healthy bones, what does it do to Harmony if your cells take calcium from the bones to neutralize the acid you have accumulated from eating too much animal protein?

HOME INSURANCE POLICY:

> *Vitamin A can protect you from gastrointestinal ulcers. If ulcer patients are more likely to develop gastrointestinal cancer, do you think Vitamin A can also reduce the incidence of this type of cancer?*

Think about this scenario: A light bulb burns out in one room of your house, and you don't have any spares on hand, so you move a lamp from another room.

You won't have any more light now than you did before; you'll just have light in a different room.

Your body works the same way. It will take whatever it needs from another place. Because you have *robbed Peter to pay Paul* you are no better off. The body is still out of balance.

You must eat more fruits and vegetables and fewer animal proteins to stabilize Harmony.

<table>
<tr><td>

HOME
INSURANCE
POLICY:

</td><td>

I have given you every plant yielding seed which is upon the face of the earth, and every tree with seed in its fruit; you shall have them for food.

- Genesis 1:29.

</td></tr>
</table>

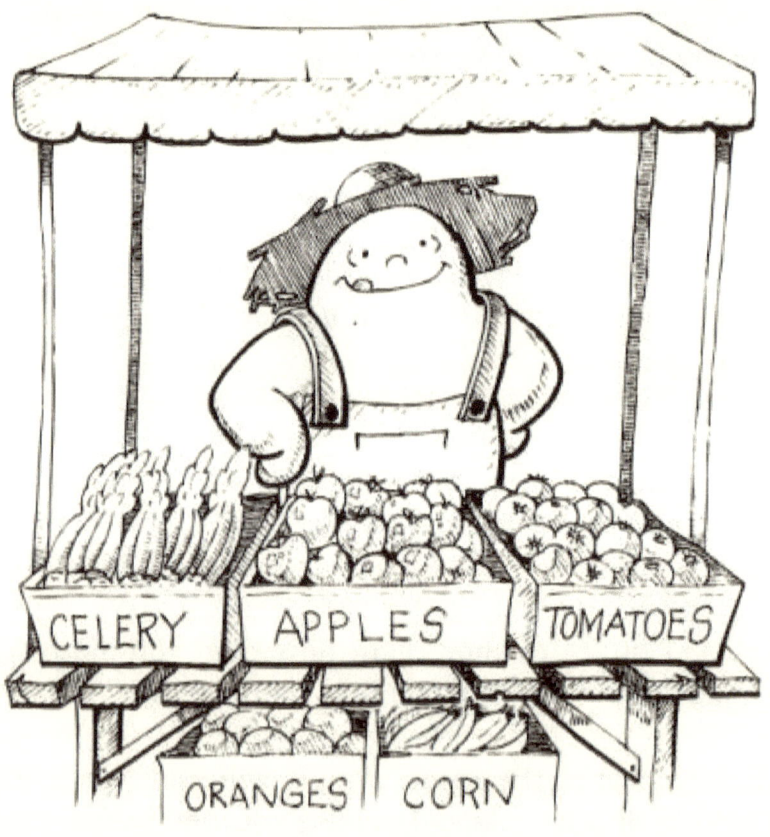

If you don't want Harmony burned by too much acid, be sure you feed fruits and vegetables to your cells.

You have now prepared the food to be used by your cells and getting it there is the job of the circulatory system. In the small intestine the blood carries on a vitally important transfer agent business. It picks up the nutrient rich food to be transported to the cells and leaves off the toxins it has collected from the cells. (In the next chapter we'll see how the cells use this food for energy.)

When you are preparing a meal in your kitchen, you will have a lot of waste. Things like egg shells, raw onion and potato peels, and cantaloupe skins are not really edible, so you throw them into the garbage disposer or trash compactor. The same thing happens in your small intestine. Since some of the food you have eaten cannot be absorbed for use by the cells, it is waste.

HOME
INSURANCE
POLICY:

> *If you bring something into the home that cannot be used, it will get in the way and clutter up your house.*

Do you know what happens if you leave garbage in the disposal for a few days and forget to turn it on?
It starts to rot.

If it sits there long enough, your whole house will smell, and you won't be able to walk in the front door without being overcome by the fumes of that rotting food. You won't want to go in the kitchen to cook, so you won't eat, and pretty soon you'll be sick.

What happens if you leave all that rubbish in your small intestine? It starts to stink up your home. Not only that. Because your *home* is so fouled, your system will no longer be able to properly prepare the food for the cells. Barred by the accumulation of garbage, the blood transfer agents will not be able to pick up nutrients, the cells won't get food, and Harmony's haven will become a disease district.

There are many health professionals who believe that a toxic colon is the primary source of disease in the body. And the longer the garbage accumulates, the greater the chance of chaos at the cellular level. Why is this?

For one thing, the typical American diet contains many unnatural chemicals—things like preservatives, food colors, refined starches, and processed foods.

These *foreign agents* are not good guests and should be asked to leave the house as soon as possible. If the colon is not strong and healthy, or the garbage does not contain enough fiber to sweep the enemy out the back door, these unwelcome guests set up housekeeping.

Then when *newcomers* arrive on the scene, they mix together and plot even more diabolical plans—for dangerous criminals like bacteria, viruses, and cancer. Or they can cause problems like constipation, diarrhea, appendicitis, or diverticulitis. When any of these conditions develop Harmony must go to *war*.

How do you keep peace on the home front? Keep the

colon clean! How can you tell if your kitchen is clean and healthy or full of foreign agents? The garbage you carry out should float in water, be large in volume and soft in consistency, easy to pass, pale color, and odorless.

In a well run kitchen, the garbage only accumulates for about 12 hours, and it is carried out on a regular basis. Many health professionals say you should eliminate after every meal, but at least once a day.

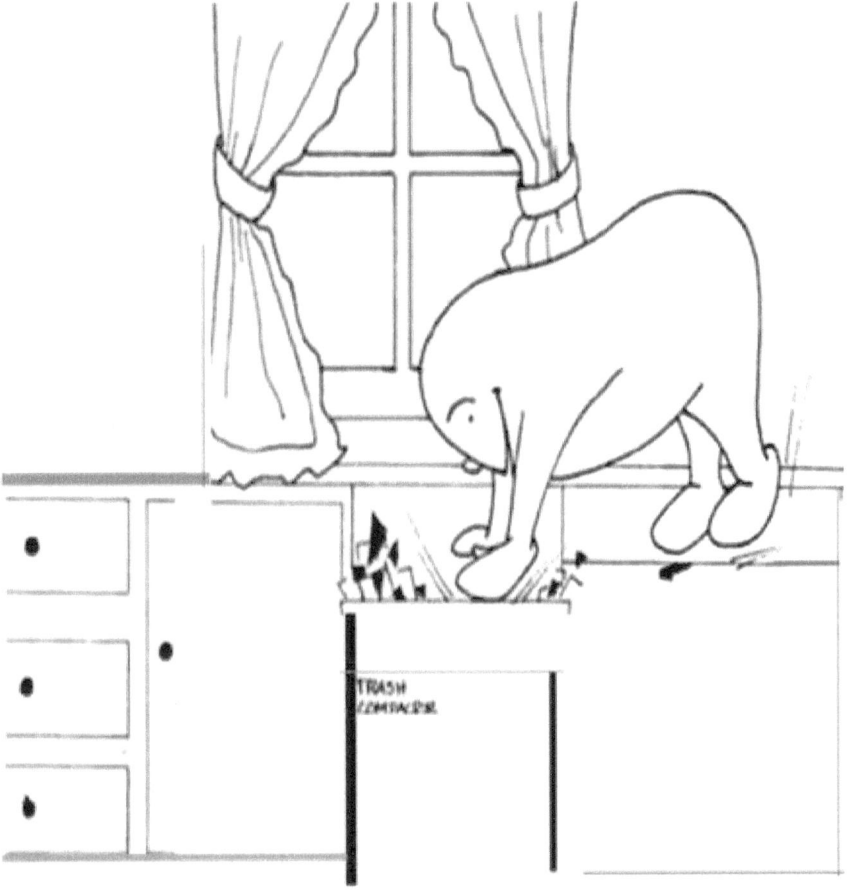

Is your kitchen clean?

What is the best way to keep your kitchen clean? Just use the FFF&E Brand of home-care products:

Foods - should be only natural and include plenty of fresh fruits and vegetables. Breads and cereals should be made of whole (live) grains.

Fluids - be sure you drink plenty of filtered or distilled water and fruit juices. Eliminate carbonated beverages and caffeine products. If you like herb teas be sure you know their effect on your body. For example, parsley tea is a good diuretic—but it can also deplete your stores of potassium.

Fiber - adds bulk to keep garbage moving through the system. By speeding up elimination, toxins do not stay in the system as long. If you have a problem with constipation, gradually increase the amount of fiber you eat. The key word here is gradually— and it may take several months for your system to make the adjustment. Remember, dietary adjustments can be a shock to your system if done too quickly.

Exercise - a brisk walk every day can increase the motility of your intestinal tract so you can keep sweeping those foreign agents out the back door.

Unfortunately, many of us have accumulated so many enemies in our kitchens that diet modification alone may not get the garbage out. In these cases, natural herb based products that have an effective but gentle effect on the colon are an excellent choice. Laxatives should be avoided because long time use can create dependency.

HOME
INSURANCE
POLICY

> *Purge me with hyssop, and I shall be clean.*
> *- Psalms 51:7*

If you want Harmony in your home, be sure that the food you prepare in your kitchen is wholesome and nutritious.

And don't forget to turn on that garbage disposal and haul out the trash as soon as the meal is finished.

Food for Thought

There is a destiny that makes us brothers
None goes his way alone;
All that we send into the lives of others,
Comes back into our own.

- Edward Markham

CHAPTER 5

The Furnace

The house has a variety of systems but none is more basic to its operation than the furnace, which burns fuel to generate the energy required to keep it warm and cozy on a cold winter night, or cool and comfortable on a hot summer afternoon.

In our model of the home/body, the furnace is the metabolism—a complex system that converts food into energy. If the furnace is going to run efficiently it is essential that it be supplied with all the right fuels in the right quantities that the cells need.

Metabolism works in two ways: it either builds up new tissue (anabolism) or breaks down tissue (catabolism). Whether it builds up or breaks down depends on the fuel it uses to generate its energy.

If the furnace in your home runs out of fuel, it will quit producing heat. If you don't give your body the right fuel, the furnace will take whatever it needs from other body parts to keep the cells running.

If your cells run out of fuel, Harmony will quit.

The life of every cell in your body depends on the fuel you supply. Without energy you have no Harmony.

The furnace in your home probably uses natural gas, propane, electricity or coal to generate heat to keep your house warm. Different types of furnaces use different types of fuel, just as each individual person requires their own particular combination of fuels—carbohydrates, proteins, and fats. When you have the right combination of fuels, you can turn it into the energy that you alone require.

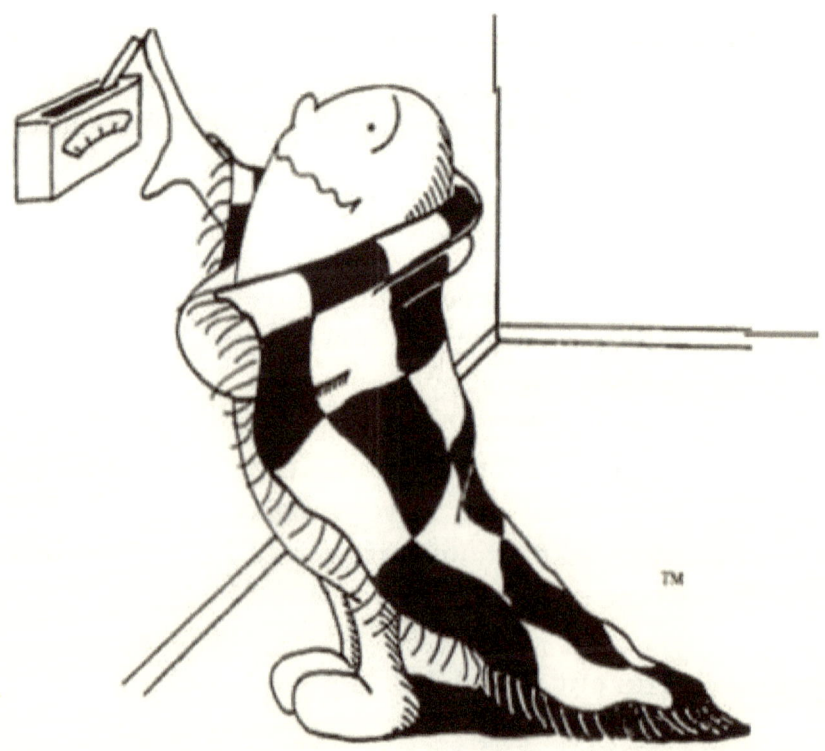

Turning food into energy is a remarkable process. How does that happen? First, let's take a look at the types of fuel your body needs, then we'll see how it uses these fuels and how much you need.

1 **Carbohydrates** are your primary source of energy and for most people 50-60 percent of the diet should come from them. We often hear carbohydrates called either *simple* or *complex.*

Simple carbohydrates are sugar-type products like ice cream, molasses, honey, and corn syrup. They are high in calories and low in vitamins and minerals, if they have any at all.

Complex carbohydrates are found in fruits, whole-grain breads, cereals, legumes, pasta, and vegetables, and there are three varieties of carbohydrates:

1. Monosaccharides are single-sugar carbs; an example of this type of sugar is blood glucose.

2. Disaccharides are two-sugar units like those found in vegetables. They are called sucrose.

3. Polysaccharides are the multiple-sugar carbohydrates. They are the starch in potatoes and similar vegetables. Cellulose, which provides fiber and roughage, is another type of polysaccharide found in plants.[32]

Since your furnace must have fuel, it converts carbohydrates into glucose—blood sugar. Please don't confuse glucose with the sweet tasting sugar found in desserts. They are not the same thing!!! Table sugar is also different from the natural sugars found in foods.

There are many of these. Two examples are fructose, which is found in fruit, and lactose, which is found in milk.

Glucose is the natural energy supply that can be used immediately by all of your cells so they can do their jobs. When a cell does not use its full serving of glucose it sends some of the leftovers back to the liver for storage. This extra glucose is turned into glycogen, which is stored in muscles where it can be used for energy. The rest of the leftovers are changed into fat and stored in fat cells. Fat cells are the components of adipose tissue.

Glucose needs a key to get into Harmony's house, and the name of the key is *insulin*. Without the hormone insulin, cells cannot get the fuel they need for energy and Harmony can't work. If the key does not fit properly, the body will develop blood sugar disorders such as diabetes and hypoglycemia.

HOME
INSURANCE
POLICY[33]

| *You need carbohydrates for a healthy diet. They are the most efficient source of energy available to your body.* — Nathaniel Lande |

❷ **Protein** is the next source of fuel for your home. It is also a predominant part of your body, being second only to water in abundance. About three-fourths of the solid part of your body is protein.[34] It is used to build cells and maintain tissues.

Proteins are also needed to build enzymes and hormones, and they are essential for the immune system. Because you can't store much protein, which may be needed in large amounts when new tissues must be built (during pregnancy, childhood growth, injury repair, infection, or surgery), you need a daily supply.

HOME INSURANCE POLICY	*Protein for the human being is built with amino acids. Every amino acid you need to build protein can be found in unprocessed foods.*

Although there are 20 amino acids, you only need to eat eight, since all the others are metabolized by your body. For many years were we taught that "vegetable foods were deficient in certain amino acids" [35] and that they were therefore considered to be incomplete sources of these vital nutrients. They were commonly called incomplete proteins.

But Dr. John A. and Mary A. McDougall say in their best-selling book, *The McDougall Plan*, that this notion was based on studies on the nutritional needs of rats done in 1914. Needless to say, the proper diet for a rat is quite different from a human's, and the McDougall's say this was proven in 1952 by Dr. William Rose.[36]

All of the essential proteins we human beings require can be found in the foods provided by our Creator. How else could our ancient ancestors have survived—do you think they knew what essential amino acids were?

HOME INSURANCE POLICY[37]	*Much of today's nutrition research is finding a strong connection between chronic disease and the excess intake of protein.*- Patrick E. Cochran

Just as dietary sugar and blood sugar are two different substances, so too are dietary proteins and physiological proteins.

What is the difference?

Physiological proteins are manufactured in the body, using carbohydrates (carbon, hydrogen, and oxygen), amino acids, nitrogen, and a few other ingredients. Since every amino acid contains nitrogen, you can readily understand that nitrogen is a vital element for our bodies. When you supply your body with the right amounts of all these nutrients it does a marvelous job of building the proteins it needs.

Dietary proteins from animals also contain nitrogen, but more than we need. Since your body is designed to eliminate moderate amounts of nitrogen as urea, in a healthy diet there is no problem.

What happens if you eat too much animal protein? There is too much excess nitrogen which is eliminated as uric acid.

Do you know what too much uric acid does? It causes gout, a painful arthritic condition.[38]

This is a very simplified explanation of what happens in your body when it has to process too much animal protein.

Can you imagine the other things that throw Harmony into chaos when you don't provide the right fuels for your body? The list is endless and unique to each individual.

HOME INSURANCE POLICY	*If you want the furnace to run efficiently, you must supply it with the right amount of carbohydrate fuel—fruits, and vegetables.*

If you really think we human beings require animal proteins, take a survey of the many, many creatures that survive and thrive on meatless diets. Among them are gorillas, horses, elephants, and cows. They manufacture their protein from the amino acids in their diets.

Americans eat too much animal protein, which has to be broken down into amino acids, and then remanufactured into useable physiological protein. Leave it to us to do it the complicated way!

What is the correct amount of protein?

Although the FDA has recently proposed 50 grams as the standard, many nutritional authorities say the average person needs about 20 to 25 grams of protein or a little less than three ounces of meat. Since Harmony can store only a limited amount of protein, the excess you eat becomes fat. And protein calories are just as fattening as carbohydrate or sugar calories.

HOME
INSURANCE
POLICY

> *A calorie is a calorie—regardless of the source: carbohydrates, fats or protein..*

3 **Fats** are the third type of fuel Harmony must have to keep the home running. Because we hear a lot about eliminating fats from our diets we may have forgotten that fats, too, are essential for good health. Besides being the taxicabs that carry vitamins A, D, E, and K to our cells, we also need fats for healthy skin and growth.

If we Americans ate normal, healthy diets, the type our Creator designed for us, fats would never have become such an issue because a good diet is naturally low in this essential component. Unfortunately, our high protein, high dairy product diets, combined with totally foreign substances like hydrogenated oils, have created heart disease, arteriosclerosis, atherosclerosis, hypertension, strokes, diabetes, and breast and colon cancers.

While news reports on cholesterol, lipoproteins, and triglycerides, monounsaturated and polyunsaturated fats are informative, heart disease still kills millions of us every year. The news may have scared you into cutting back on fats, but do you really understand how it works in your body?

There are two types of fats: saturated and unsaturated. These terms refer to the structure of fatty acids, which are the main ingredients of fats. In order to use fats, the body metabolizes them into these fatty acids, which produce twice as much energy per gram than either carbohydrates or protein. (Fats = 9kcal. per gram; protein and carbohydrates = 4kcal. per gram. Kcal. is the scientific name for kilocalories, commonly called calories.)

HOME INSURANCE POLICY	*Two much of one element =* *out of balance on two or more.*

You can visualize fatty acids as a motorcade. Each car is a carbon atom and each car can hold a certain number of passengers. The passengers are hydrogen atoms. When the car is full of passengers, it is saturated.

What happens when two cars are empty, but they continue along right next to each other in the motorcade?

They are unsaturated—just like unsaturated fats. Monounsaturated fats do not have hydrogen atoms attached to them. If a lot of empty cars are traveling together, you will have polyunsaturated fats. When you mix these three types of motorcades you have triglycerides: saturated, monounsaturated, and polyunsaturated fats. It is the saturated fat that wrecks Harmony and creates havoc in your body. Do you know why that happens?

HOME INSURANCE POLICY

Although dietary fats are concentrated energy, they are also concentrated danger.

Cholesterol, another fat-like substance, gets the blame. It joins the motorcade because, like fatty acids, it is essential to good health. It is also necessary for production of hormones, cellular structure, and metabolism. In fact, cholesterol is so essential that our livers produce what we need. Unfortunately, we add to this natural supply by ingesting more fat. In fact, we eat so much fat that our body's production is only about sixty to seventy-five percent of what we have in our blood!

Do you know what happens to all those fats in your blood stream?

Pretend that your triglycerides and cholesterol motorcades have arrived at a river, and need a ferry to reach their destination in the cells. They call up the liver, which manufactures a very special ferry called lipoproteins. The cholesterol and triglycerides jump on board the VLDL (very low density lipoproteins) which is now in the blood for the ride through the arteries. The first stop is the muscle and fat cells, where the triglycerides disembark. Muscle cells use this fat for immediate energy but the fat cells store it for future use.

HOME INSURANCE POLICY	*Your body manufactures the amount of cholesterol it needs. Don't throw Harmony into chaos by overloading on dietary fats.*

Alone on the ferry (now called LDL) cholesterol continues its journey, giving these essential nutrients to each cell asking for a donation. If the ferry boat is overloaded with cholesterol, some of its cargo spills overboard, and attaches to the walls of the arteries. But your body is so astonishing that it makes another ferry (HDL - high density lipoproteins) that comes along to pick up this mess and take it back to the liver. At the liver it is either reprocessed or eliminated.

You can remember LDL and HDL this way:

L = Lousy or Lethal;
H = Happy or Healthy!

As advanced as we are in the scientific and medical communities, we still don't know for sure how all this gets accomplished. But your body does exactly what needs to be done.

When there is too much cholesterol, or too little HDL, the blood stream is overloaded and starts to thicken. Cholesterol hangs onto the walls of the arteries, and loads them up with fat. You now have atherosclerosis. If you don't clean up your act and eliminate excess fat from your diet, excess calcium, which also circulates in the blood, will penetrate the cholesterol plaque and harden the arteries. You now have arteriosclerosis.

HOME
INSURANCE
POLICY

> *When we choose fatty foods for taste and texture, Harmony pays dearly for our choice.*

Now that we have reviewed the three sources of fuel for Harmony—carbohydrates, proteins, and fat—you'll probably want to know how Harmony uses this fuel.

Glucose (blood sugar) is delivered to the cell, and once inside it is transported to Harmony's fireplace—the mitochondria—where it is burned. This process leaves *ash* in the cell that must be disposed of. If the kitchen has sent too many acid type foods to burn, Harmony will have acid ash.

Typical acid producing foods are dairy products, grains, fish, meats and poultry. Fruits and vegetables leave an alkaline ash.

Since your cells are designed to work in a slightly alkaline atmosphere, which foods do you think Harmony will prefer?

HOME
INSURANCE
POLICY

> *When your cells are working in acid they may as well be swimming upstream.*

Do you know why it is necessary to understand the difference between acid ash and alkaline ash foods?

To maintain a state of wellness for Harmony, you must enable your cells to build themselves up. This work is done by the enzymes, which can only do their job in an alkaline environment. Building up and restoring cells is an anabolic process. It is good for Harmony and it is essential for your health.

When the cellular enzymes have to work in acid, their activity level is either slowed down or halted altogether. When this happens, Harmony starves and the cell dies. This is called catabolism—and it is the huge front door that allow diseases and degenerative disorders to enter your home. Your stomach is the only organ designed to work with acid.

What else creates acidity in the body?

Stress is a major producer of acid. Many times the end result of stress is too much stomach acid and you end up with an ulcer.
Exercise also creates acid. Have you ever felt the pain of lactic acid build-up in your muscles while you were doing strenuous exercises?

This happens when the body does not have enough oxygen to use its regular fuel so it breaks up other energy elements that can burn without oxygen. As you know if you have experienced lactic acid build-up, the muscles will shut down very quickly with this acid diet.

Some other effects of too much acid are morning stiffness, anxiety, tension, and nervousness.

So how do you protect your home from the damage caused by acid-producing high protein foods, stress, and exercise?

Eat more fruits and vegetables and stock your pantry with alkaline forming minerals like calcium, magnesium, potassium, and sodium. These minerals will actually buffer the acid and help bring your pH back into balance.

And what is pH?

That is an abbreviation for the phrase *Potential of Hydrogen.* pH is a measure of the amount of acidity or alkalinity in a substance in a range from 1 to 15.

If the substance is neutral, like water, it will have a pH of 7. Numbers 1 through 6 are measures of acidity and numbers 8 through 15 measure alkalinity. A cola drink usually has a reading of 2.5—so it is very acid. In fact, you would have to drink about 35 glasses of water at a pH of 10 to neutralize the acid in one cola drink!

HOME INSURANCE POLICY	*Your blood pH must remain between 7.35 and 7.45. Too much shift either way can be fatal.*

Since many, many diseases require an acid atmosphere, you can see why the guests you invite in your front door have a direct relationship on the health and Harmony of your home.

A discussion about fuel for Harmony's furnace would not be complete without a look at quantity.

How much fuel does your home need?

As we have already said, energy is measured in calories, or kilocalories to be precise. Your calorie consumption should be based not only on your age, ideal weight and height, but also take into consideration the amount of energy you expend for activities as well as your general fat/muscle ratio.

A very lean, muscular person who weighs 200 pounds will need more calories to maintain their weight than a person with a high percentage of body fat.

Why is that?

Because muscle tissues use more calories than adipose (fat) tissues. Muscle tissue also weighs more but has less volume.

How fast your body burns calories is measured by the Basal Metabolic Rate (BMR). This rate is calculated as the amount of energy you expend while resting just to perform the basic, life-sustaining functions such as breathing, digestion, and heart beat. Added to the basal metabolic rate would be the amount of energy you require for exercise.

After you have figured your daily need for calories, you can easily determine your carbohydrate, protein and fat requirements. Although recommended quantities vary from one nutritional expert to another, the following amounts are averages compiled from a number of diets. (See Appendix.)

Carbohydrates:

Approximately <u>61 percent</u> of your calories should be spent on this basic fuel—most of these should come from complex carbohydrates.

Fats:

Use no more than <u>23 percent</u> of your daily calories for fat—with the majority being unsaturated fat. If you have high cholesterol, your recommended allowance of fat could be as low as 11 percent.

Proteins:

The final <u>16 percent</u> of your dietary calories should be proteins—some diets go as high as 23 percent protein.

To summarize the nutritional requirements to keep Harmony's furnace running at peak efficiency, here is a simple formula for you:

A Simple Formula for Nutrition

Carbohydrates	=	Glucose	⎤
Proteins	=	Amino Acids	+ Oxygen + Enzymes = Energy
Fat	=	Fatty Acids	⎦ ↑

Vitamins
&
Minerals

Now, let's look at another theory about healthy fuel for your furnace. Have you ever heard of *Food Combining*? This is a complex subject, but here are a few basics for you to consider:

❶ Fruits digest faster than any other food (approximately 20 minutes) and therefore should be eaten alone—otherwise they can be *over-cooked* in the stomach and cause gastric distress.

❷ Vegetables can be eaten with any food (other than fruit), but dairy products, starches, and grains and nuts are digested better if not mixed with one another.

Sweet Fruits, Melons, Tart Fruits:
Eat these alone.

Vegetables and salads:
Eat with any <u>one</u> of these:
Dairy products, Starches,
Meats and Nuts

"So many rules for food combining have developed that people become overwhelmed and lose sight of the fact that individuals have to develop their own from direct experiences. The simplest rule of food combining is to eat foods or combinations of foods that in our direct experience are easiest to digest."

- Gabriel Cousens, M.D.,
Spiritual Nutrition and The Rainbow Diet" [39]

How many carbohydrates, proteins and fats do you need for Harmony?

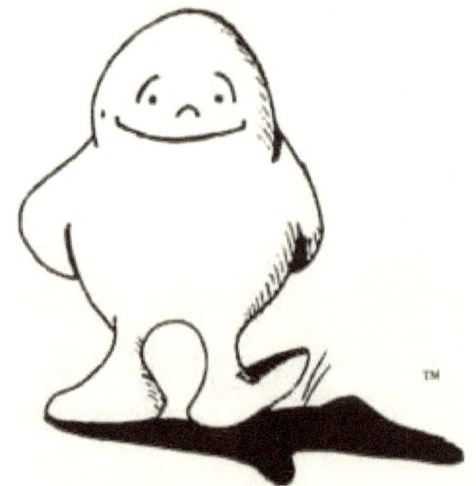

CHAPTER 6

The Pantry

Well organized homes have a pantry—a storage place for food items to feed and maintain the family.

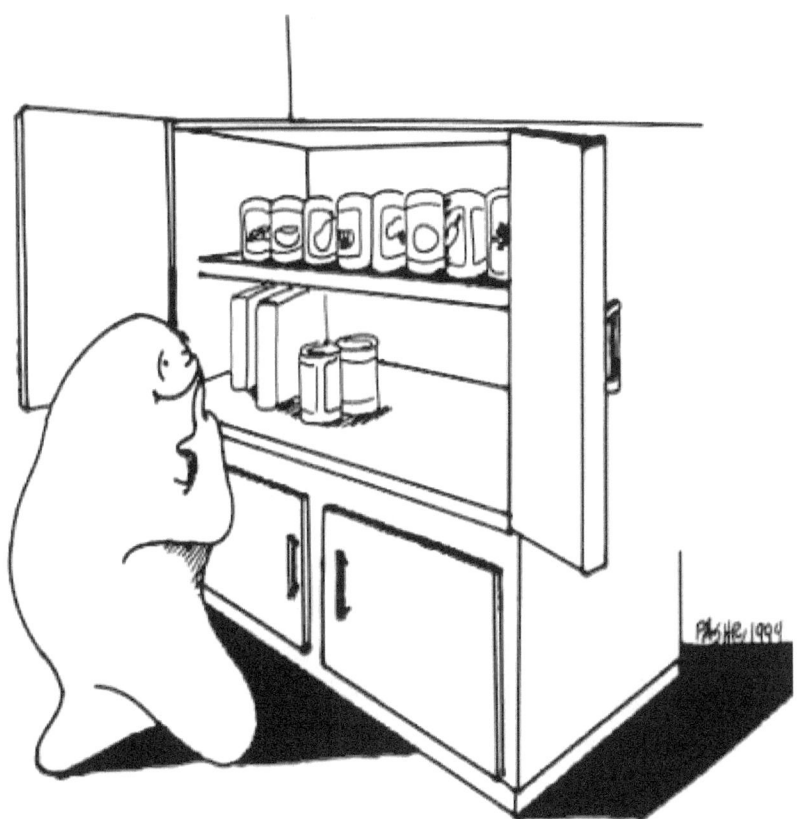

In a well stocked pantry you might find things like whole grain cereals, boxes of iron rich raisins, brown rice, unbleached flour, whole wheat bread, organically grown potatoes, beans, nuts, etc.

If you want to keep Harmony in peak operating condition, it is important that you supply essential nutrients like vitamins, minerals, amino acids, and enzymes. Let's set aside one shelf for each of these items and see what a well stocked pantry for Harmony should contain.

HOME
INSURANCE
POLICY

> *Some vitamins and minerals work together like soap and water. Others complement, like salt and pepper. Still others can throw Harmony out of balance - like turning on the heater and air conditioner at the same time.*

FIRST SHELF: Enzymes

Enzymes are first. They are required for everything your miraculous body does—seeing, thinking, smelling, breathing, tasting, talking, playing and walking, to name just a few. You can't have life without enzymes because they are in every living thing. Most of your enzymes are manufactured in your body by the proteins. There are two types of enzymes: metabolic and digestive.

Metabolic enzymes run the body and make repairs. Digestive enzymes help you process carbohydrates and fat and turn them into fuel your body can use.

A third type of enzyme is found in raw foods. They start food digestion and help the body's own digestive enzymes so they don't have to work so hard.

Enzymes, which are really sophisticated proteins, won't work by themselves. They need help from vitamins or minerals to get their jobs done.

<table>
<tr><td>HOME
INSURANCE
POLICY</td><td>*Digestive enzymes are the strongest enzymes in your body. You can't digest your food without them.*</td></tr>
</table>

SECOND SHELF: Vitamins

Vitamins—Harmony's Helpers—are on the next shelf. Vitamins help convert food into energy and help manufacture blood cells. As chief assistants to enzymes they help activate the never ending chain of chemical reactions in our bodies. Healthy cells cannot be maintained without vitamins.

There are two types of vitamins: fat soluble and water soluble.

The fat soluble vitamins (A, D, E, and K) can be stored in body fat and used later. If too many of these are accumulated in body tissues they may create toxic effects.

The water soluble vitamins are the eight Bs and C. Because they dissolve in body fluids, excesses are eliminated by urine or sweat.

HOME INSURANCE POLICY	*Without vitamins, your immune system cannot keep unwelcomed guests out of your house. You are opening the door and inviting disease in for a visit.*

In 1943, the U.S. Government recommended that certain amounts of vitamins be included in food served to the Armed Forces. These RDAs (Recommended Dietary Allowances) are updated every five years and indicate only the average amounts needed by healthy people to prevent deficiency diseases. For optimum health many nutritional experts recommend quantities much higher than the RDAs.

If you have a chronic disease, infection, or cancer, if you smoke, drink alcohol, take certain vitamin depleting medications, or have excessive stress (either emotional or environmental) in your life, you could require a lot more vitamins than the RDA.

Elderly people, dieters, pregnant or lactating women, and people recovering from surgery should supplement their diets with extra vitamins. Athletically active people may also need more vitamins since they tend to eat more carbohydrates, which increases the need for thiamine, and sweating causes excretion of some essential nutrients.[40]

HOME
INSURANCE
POLICY

> *Enzymes are lazy. They don't get to work until vitamins and minerals come along and give them a kick.*

A well-stocked vitamin inventory for Harmony would include these:

Vitamin A - builds immune response, keeps mucous membranes moist; important for growth and healthy skin; deficiency causes night blindness. It is toxic in large doses. Found in beta-carotene, a component of carrots, as well as broccoli and spinach.

Vitamin B-1 - Thiamine - is beneficial to nervous system; promotes growth in children, strengthens immune system, assists in metabolizing carbohydrates. Deficiency causes fatigue, insomnia. Found in asparagus, brown rice, brewer's yeast, beans, whole grains, nuts and seeds, and wheat germ.

Vitamin B-2 - Riboflavin - necessary for energy production, this vitamin is frequently lacking in American diets. Necessary for the eyes and healthy skin. Found in almonds, brewer's yeast, broccoli, leafy green vegetables, yogurt, wild rice, and mushrooms.

Vitamin B-3 - Niacin - is required by many body systems including digestion, production of energy, metabolizing cholesterol, sex hormone synthesis, skin and nerves. Deficiency leads to skin problems, headaches, possible high blood pressure, mental problems. Found in almonds, avocados, bananas, brewer's yeast, legumes, and whole grains.

Vitamin B-5 - Pantothenic Acid - is needed by adrenal glands for cortisone production to prevent arthritis and high cholesterol. Builds antibodies, fights stress and nerve disorders. Deficiency causes anemia. Found in brown rice, brewer's yeast, broccoli, legumes, yams, and whole grains.

Vitamin B-6 - Pyridoxine - essential for red blood cells, amino acids and metabolism, healthy skin and nerves. Important immune stimulant. Deficiency causes depression, anemia, and skin lesions. Found in avocados, bananas, brewer's yeast, buckwheat, legumes, and nuts.

Vitamin B-12 - Cyano Cobalamin - vital for proper functioning of central nervous system and red blood cell formation. Deficiency can cause paralysis and death but symptoms of depletion may not appear for five years since it is stored in the body. B-12 is synthesized in the body but is also found in yeast grown on a B-12 medium, spirulina and soy sauce.

Biotin - is a member of the B-complex vitamin family. It is needed for amino acid and essential fatty acid metabolism. Deficiency results in skin and muscle problems. Found in brewer's yeast, grapefruit, raspberries, and tomatoes

Choline - another member of the B-complex; necessary for proper brain and neurotransmitter functioning.

Effective as treatment for Alzheimer's and nervous system disorders. Found in unrefined vegetable oils, legumes, and soy products.

<table>
<tr><td>HOME
INSURANCE
POLICY</td><td>*Millions of Americans are hospitalized each year for adverse reactions to drugs. Unlike vitamins and minerals, drugs are not natural.*</td></tr>
</table>

Folic Acid - a B-Complex component, is required for production of DNA, blood, enzyme efficiency, and vital for new cells. Deficiency creates digestive system problems. Found in brewer's yeast, broccoli, soy products, and leafy green vegetables.

Inositol - another member of the B-complex family but not a vitamin. It works with biotin and choline; lowers cholesterol and controls fatty deposits. Aids in control of diabetic complications. Found in almonds, beans, oranges, onions, peanut butter, oats, peas, tomatoes, and zucchini.

PABA - Para-Aminobenzoic Acid - also a B-complex family member and component of folic acid. Is effective as a sun screen and treatment of burns and vitiligo. Found in brewer's yeast, molasses and wheat germ.

Vitamin C - Ascorbic Acid - is essential for the immune system and forming new collagen. Works as an anti-oxidant to fight free radicals. Speeds healing, effective in treating colds and other viruses, and lowering cholesterol. Found in citrus fruits, green peppers, papaya, tomatoes, potatoes, greens, kiwi, cauliflower and broccoli.

Bioflavonoids - are part of the C complex and help it function. They are also effective in preventing hardening of the arteries and enhance strength of the circulatory system (blood vessels, veins, and capillaries). Bioflavonoids protect connective tissues, help lower cholesterol, and stimulate bile production. Because the body does not manufacture its own supply of this nutrient, it is important to get it in supplements and food sources such as buckwheat, most vegetables, and the white inside of citrus fruit skins.

Vitamin D - can be synthesized by the body from sunlight. Working with Vitamin A it utilizes phosphorus and calcium to build bones and teeth. Effective in treating eye problems and protects against colon cancer. Found in cod liver oil.

Vitamin E - Tocopherol - stimulates the immune system and retards cellular aging. Improves skin and works with selenium to fight free radicals. Deficiency results in nerve and muscle degeneration and anemia. Found in almonds, leafy vegetables, soy products, wheat germ, beans and peas.

Vitamin K - is essential for blood clotting. Helps heal broken blood vessels in the eye and prevents bone loss. Metabolized normally in the intestinal tract, it can be eaten in leafy green vegetables, potatoes, bran, yogurt, and tomatoes.

RNA - Ribonucleic Acid - a natural substance that is thought to be an important ingredient in the brain's chemistry and is nicknamed the "memory molecule." [41] Also helps improve skin tone and appearance. Found in yeast.

HOME INSURANCE POLICY[42]

> *No longer are advocates of better nutrition dismissed as food faddists and health-food nuts. The evidence is already in that how we eat has a direct bearing on how healthy or sick we are.*
> - Nathaniel Lande

THIRD SHELF: Minerals

Minerals—your precious metals—are the next item you need to stock in Harmony's pantry. It won't matter how much gold and silver you have stored in your bank vault if you don't have enough copper, calcium, chromium, magnesium, and zinc in your pantry for Harmony.

Like vitamins, minerals are needed to jump start the enzymes—they just don't get going without mineral aid. Minerals unite nutrients with Harmony, the way mortar holds the bricks on your house together.

They also keep the body pH in balance, making sure that it is alkaline and not acid. Minerals transport oxygen, regulate the beating of your heart, help form bones, digest food, keep your furnace (metabolism) running, and assist in balancing you mentally and emotionally.

HOME
INSURANCE
POLICY[43]

> *The difference between vitamins and minerals: Minerals are "in" organic compounds; vitamins "are" organic compounds.*
>
> - Nathaniel Lande

There are two groups of minerals. The *essential* minerals are calcium, magnesium, and phosphorus. The *trace* minerals are copper, chromium, iron, iodine, manganese, potassium, selenium, and zinc. Minerals are all over the body, but their main home is bone and muscle tissue.

Essential Minerals:

Calcium is necessary for strong bones and teeth, and is especially important in growing children, pregnant women, and elderly people. It is the most abundant mineral in your body—you have about two and a half pounds (1,200 grams). The Framingham Heart Study discovered that men who ate higher levels of calcium had a lower risk for developing hypertension.[44] Source?
Leafy vegetables.

Magnesium works with calcium for teeth and bone formation. It is also important for muscles and nerve function. Source? Peanuts, beans, and whole grains to get this mineral.

Phosphorus is the third essential for bones and teeth. It is also needed to get oxygen to the brain, for proper cell growth and nervous system function. About one percent of your weight is phosphorus. Source? It is found in many, many foods and we usually have enough in our diets.

Trace Minerals:

Copper helps in your iron absorption, protein metabolism, bone mineralization, blood clotting and formation. Source? Raisins, sea vegetation such as kelp, high fiber cereals, nuts, and legumes.

Chromium is essential, even in trace amounts, for proper glucose regulation. Nutritionists recommend 200 to 600 mcg daily, but the average American only gets about 25 mcg in their diet. People are supplementing their diets with chromium picolinate and chromium polynicotinate acid. Exercise increases the need for chromium supplementation. Source? Brewer's yeast, honey, whole grains, grapes, and raisins.

Iron has to join proteins and copper to make hemoglobin, the messengers that carry oxygen to Harmony. Without sufficient iron the tissues become starved for oxygen and you feel tired. But too much iron can be very toxic, especially in children, who can be innocently killed by iron overdoses when they eat iron supplements[45] intended for adults. Source? Leafy green vegetables, prunes, legumes, and whole grains will give you iron.

Iodine is necessary for proper thyroid function and metabolism, healthy hair, skin, and nails. Source? Sea vegetables.

Manganese nourishes the brain and nerves. It also helps metabolize fats and sugar. Manganese supplements should be taken under the guidance of a health professional as high levels can cause a person to become violent. Source? Bananas, pineapple, green vegetables, whole grains, nuts, and cereals.

Potassium is very popular with Harmony, and your cells have more of this mineral than any other. It is needed for proper nerve function and helps maintain the amount of fluid in your cells. Heart patients or people taking diuretics may need potassium supplements, but increasing consumption should only be done under guidance of a health professional. Because it must be in balance with sodium, too much sodium from processed foods can increase the need for potassium. There is no RDA for this mineral. Source? Fresh foods and legumes.

Selenium works with vitamins A and C to produce an anti-oxidant effect and fight free radicals. Source? Sea kelp, garlic, brewer's yeast, wheat germ, and sesame seeds.

Zinc is vital for proper immune system performance and development of insulin. Because of its effect on the brain, it can be effective in the treatment of nerve related disorders. Zinc is also important for healthy hair and skin. Do not take zinc supplements for long periods of time because it must be in balance with copper. If zinc is needed, a health professional should monitor your supplementation program. Source? Mushrooms, brewer's yeast, and wheat germ.

HOME
INSURANCE
POLICY

> *Disease prevention and treatment both start with*
> *sound nutrition.*

You must eat foods that contain minerals since Harmony cannot manufacture (synthesize) them. Because minerals make up four percent of your body weight, you can see how important they are.

If you weigh 150 pounds, you should have six pounds of these precious metals in your pantry to keep Harmony well.

HOME
INSURANCE
POLICY[46]

> *A nutrient deficiency can be caused by lack of*
> *absorption. If your body can't make what you*
> *need, take what you need.* -Linda Rector-Page

FOURTH SHELF: Amino Acids

Amino acids - the builders of protein - are the next item in Harmony's pantry. Some of the amino acids are formed naturally in the body. They are labeled *non-essential* since you don't have to consume them because your splendid body manufactures them. The other group is called *essential* because the body cannot create them; therefore, you must get them from food.

Semi-essential amino acids are partially created in the body, and the balance of them must come from food.

Vegetables contain many of the essential amino acids and you should feed Harmony a variety of them to provide your cells with these nutrients which you need for growth, maintenance and repair[47] of Harmony. Check with your health professional if you think you need amino acid supplements.

HOME INSURANCE POLICY[48]	*Carnitine stimulates enzymes to help regulate metabolism of fat, provides energy to the heart muscle, and increases oxidation of fat for weight loss and energy.*

With all these nutrients in your pantry, you can have Harmony in your home.

CHAPTER 7

The Telephone

We use the telephone to communicate with others anywhere in the world. If you live in Atlanta and want to talk to Aunt Mary in Maine, all you have to do is pick up your cell phone and dial a number.

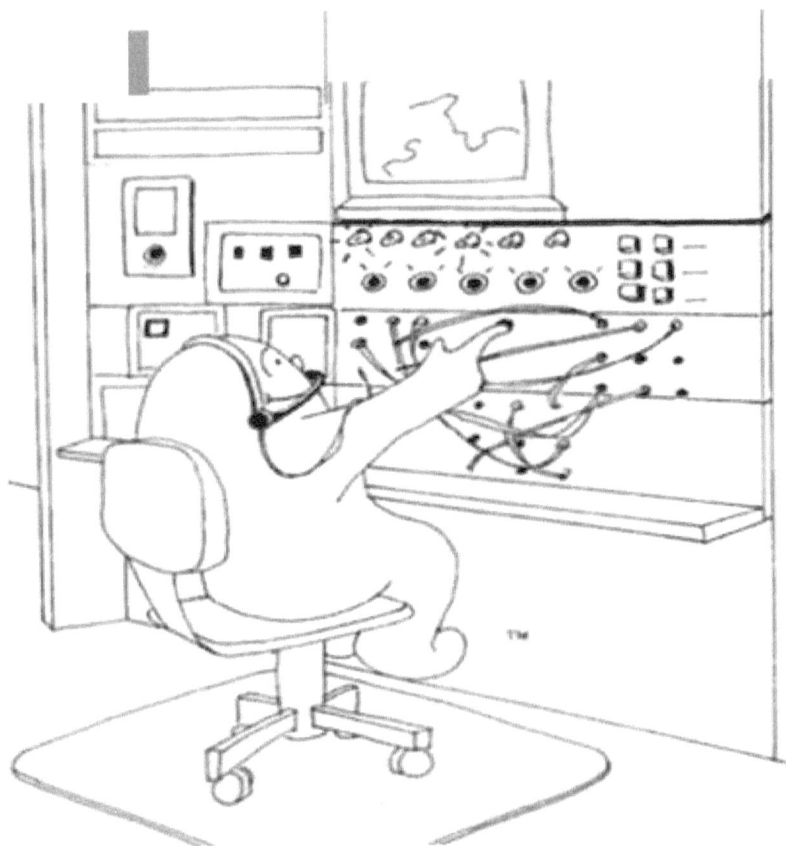

Your brain is your communication with Harmony.

With our modern phone system we can send and receive messages, store them in a data bank, or retrieve and erase them.

Your extraordinary brain is like the telephone. It is your central communication system. Every chore done by your home/body involves the nervous system. The message *get to work* must be delivered from the brain, through the spinal cord, to all the cells involved—whether it is something visible and controllable like blinking the eyes, or completely involuntary, like digesting food or breathing.

What happens if you want to call Aunt Mary and the cell phone towers are down? Your call can't get through. Likewise, without proper nutrition and maintenance, we jeopardize the only means we have of conveying information from our brain to the cells in its network.

Unlike the phone company, which only has about a billion customers, your brain can send and receive messages from all seventy-five trillion cells in your incredible network. That's an awesome number of clients!

To keep up with this very high-volume of data communication, the brain has more than 100 billion sophisticated operators called neuron cells. Each of these neurons can carry on 10,000 conversations at one time if necessary.

(Is it any wonder then that we have never been able to develop a computer that can equal the human brain?)

Do you know what this chatter is all about?

What's going on in your home that requires such an extensive messaging system?

And how do messages get carried from one place in the body to another?

HOME INSURANCE POLICY	*While enormous strides have been made in communications in recent years, there's still a lot to be said for the smile.* - Franklin P. Jones

With a phone in your house, you can swap information with anyone in the world. Your boss can call and tell you what time to be at the office. Your friends can text you what time they will arrive at the airport so you can pick them up. Your spouse can let you know where to meet them after work. Your kids can ask you to pick them up from school. Your parents can let you know what time you are expected for dinner. And on and on.

How would you function without your cell phone?

In a similar way, every activity in your body is organized and communicated to by the brain: breathing and blinking; circulation, digestion and elimination; growth and reproduction; feeling, seeing, tasting, and hearing; learning and thinking; going to sleep and waking up, to name a few. Everything is under the control of the brain.

The brain and central nervous system are an extremely complex system. We've already told you about the operators—those wondrous neurons. But they can't do all the work by themselves. They have many helpers. They also have various supervisors that tell them what to do.

The helpers are glial cells and they outnumber neurons about five or ten to one. That's a lot of brain cells! Some glial cells are called astrocytes. By using an electrochemical process, they interact with the neurons to carry on all those conversations.

The other glial cells are called oligodendrocytes. They form the myelin covering on the axons—the tentacles of the neuron. This myelin is sometimes called the white matter since it is a sort of whitish color.

You've probably heard of gray matter.

Do you know what it is?

Gray matter is the surface of the cerebrum, and it is called the cerebral cortex. It stores all of your long-term memory.

People who are smart may be told that they have a lot of gray matter, meaning that they store a lot of information. It does not mean that they actually have more brain than anyone else.

HOME
INSURANCE
POLICY

> *There is no problem that we cannot solve if we*
> *can corral our resources behind it.*
>   - Coretta Scott King

Because every life experience is recorded in your brain it needs plenty of storage space. That's why the surface is folded and crumpled with ridges and valleys like a piece of crinkled up paper—there's lots of surface to the cerebral cortex crammed under your skull.

The cerebral cortex gives us the ability to speak and write as well as to think and solve problems. It also provides us with imagination.

Short-term memory is stored in the middle of the brain. If a person has a stroke or other brain damaging disease that injures the inner part, they may not be able to remember what they ate for breakfast and yet may have perfect recollection of their five-year old birthday party.

Do you have a personal computer?

Short term memory would be like the data you have typed, and can read on the monitor, but have not yet stored. Until the data is transferred to the hard drive, or a floppy disk, if there is a power failure you could easily lose all that information.

Long-term memory is like the hard drive on your computer. It stores the information for later retrieval—even years later.

Brain surgery is as old as Stone Age man, who performed the first skull opening operations about 12,000 years ago.

Because there is so much work to be supervised by the brain and such a vast number of messages to be delivered, many of these activities are done automatically and you don't even have to think about it. Your heart beats, your lungs breathe, and food is digested; your kidneys eliminate toxins, the blood is circulated, and hormones are produced.

This vital work is done by a team, the autonomic nervous system and the endocrine system. They each have a different method of transmitting information and getting their share of the work done.

The autonomic nervous system sends brief messages by electrical impulse. Because they are transmitted very quickly—over 600 feet per second—they get an immediate response.

Your autonomic nervous system has two divisions, the sympathetic and the parasympathetic. The sympathetic nervous system reacts to all your immediate needs—like jerking your hand away from something hot.

After you get the adrenalin rush generated by the sympathetic system, the parasympathetic kicks in to calm you down.

Have you ever known anyone who was energetic or hyperactive?

Or anyone too laid back?

The hyperactive person is dominated by their sympathetic system whereas the lazy or laid back person is controlled by the parasympathetic system. Either way, they are out of balance.

The endocrine system generally works more slowly. It is supervised by the hypothalamus. The hypothalamus is assisted by the pituitary gland. The endocrine laborers are ductless glands and include the adrenals, pancreas, thyroid and parathyroid, thymus, ovaries, and testes. Working together they maintain Harmony's environment.

These laborers manufacture hormones—each one making its own brand. These hormones are used to send messages through the blood stream. It may take days to make a delivery but the information has a more lasting effect once it is received by the cell.

Do you know what messages the endocrine system transmits?

You're probably most familiar with the fastest endocrine messenger, the adrenal glands. When your home is in danger, the adrenals send a message that prepares you to take action to protect it—what some call the *fight or flight* response.

Other endocrine commands come from the thyroid, which tells the metabolism how fast to run, the pancreas, which controls insulin, and the parathyroid, which regulates the amount of calcium in the blood.

By now you are probably wondering what all this has to do with wellness.

How in the world can you possibly affect this marvelous operation?

Your brain uses one-fourth of the energy required by your total body. That is an astounding amount of fuel.

HOME INSURANCE POLICY	*Brain cells are pigs - they consume one-fourth of the fuel you put in your body, and use one-fifth of the body's blood supply.*

Glucose is the brain's primary source of energy, and this fuel is used to produce about 20 of the 200 hormones manufactured in your body. It is also used to transmit all those messages to each of those 75 trillion clients many times every day.

The brain also needs amino acids. Proteins you eat are broken down into amino acids in the intestinal tract and shipped to the brain where they are used to manufacture chemicals called neurotransmitters.

HOME
INSURANCE
POLICY

> *Protein is brain food but eating more
> of it won't make you smarter - just fatter.*

How do those 100 billion operators handle all those conversations?

Did you ever play the game called Gossip when you were a child?

You'd sit in a circle with a group of friends and one would whisper a secret to the person next to them. The person who heard the secret would pass it on to the next, and so it would go until the private message was finally passed on to the person who started it.

Your neurons work in a similar way. One neuron receives a message from one of the 75 trillion cells in your body, and it passes it on to the next neuron. When you whisper in the ear of the person next to you playing Gossip, you don't have to actually touch them in order for them to hear what you say. Neurons also pass messages along without actually touching.

HOME
INSURANCE
POLICY[50]

> *Cells live and die by the constant chatter
> streaming through their interiors...*
>> Shannon Brownlee,
>> U.S. News & World Report

The message is sort of like an internal Morse Code. It goes over the wires (the axons) as an electrical impulse. When it gets to the end of the wire (this is called the dendrite), a chemical called a neurotransmitter picks up the message and takes it to the dendrites of the next neuron. This alters the electrical energy in the receiving cell, so it takes the message and passes it on to the next neuron, also using neurotransmitters to bridge the gap. This gap is called the synapse.

Have you ever driven your car across a draw bridge?

If the bridge is opened when you arrive, and the operator is not there to close the bridge, you can't get across the water, can you?

Neurotransmitters are like the draw bridge. Your message can't cross from one neuron to the next without the neurotransmitters. Your diet must have the right nutrients if you want your brain to manufacture its neurotransmitters.

HOME
INSURANCE
POLICY

> *Neurotransmitters are like a draw bridge—you can't get your message across without them.*

When you play Gossip, the message may start out with an instruction: *Go in the kitchen and get a glass of milk and bring it to me.* By the time the message is passed from friend to friend to friend in the circle, it may come back as something entirely different: *Go in the backyard and get the kittens and take them to my mom.*

This may seem like a simple comparison, but that's what can go wrong in your brain if the messages are not correctly received and transmitted from cell to cell.

For example, the neurotransmitter *acetylcholine* is needed for proper transmission of thoughts. Without it, you may develop Alzheimer's disease. You may tell a person with Alzheimer's to pour a glass of milk, but because their messaging system is either skewed with faulty neurotransmitters, or possibly has none at all, they will go in the back yard and get the kittens.

Choline is needed for the manufacture of the neurotransmitter acetylcholine. Although the body synthesizes choline, lecithin is a good natural source.

Don't you think Alzheimer's patients could be helped with the proper nutrients? New research seems to indicate that they can.

What are some of the other neurotransmitters your brain needs and what sort of messages do they carry?

Two significant brain chemicals are serotonin and norepinephrine. A lack of either one can cause depression. The amino acid tryptophan is an essential component of serotonin. Tyrosine, another amino acid, is used in the manufacture of dopamine. Since amino acids come from proteins, you can see that protein is an essential component of your brain's wellness?

Do you know what other nutrients are essential for Harmony's communication system?

- **Pantothenic acid** is also required for production of acetylcholine as well as the neurotransmitter sphingosine.

- **RNA** (ribonucleic acid) has been nicknamed the *memory molecule*[51] since it is involved with memory and learning. RNA is found in yeast.

- **Folic acid** deficiency can lead to mental problems (depression, schizophrenia, and dementia). Derivatives of this nutrient are coenzymes for neurotransmitters. Folic acid can be effective in reducing neural tube (open spine) defects if the mother is taking it at the time of conception.

HOME
INSURANCE
POLICY

> *B" is for Brain - and Vitamin B.*

- **Vitamin B-1** (Thiamin) is essential for carbohydrate metabolism, and nervous system cells are sensitive to this process. For that reason, the nerves and brain need adequate supplies of this vitamin.

- **Vitamin B-2** (Riboflavin) is absolutely essential for healthy eyes. If your eyes are sensitive to light (photophobia), you should find out if you have a B-2 deficiency. Without enough of this vitamin you can become moody, depressed, and irritable.

- **Vitamin B-3** (Niacin) is another co-enzyme required if Harmony is to have a healthy nervous system. Without sufficient quantities, emotional problems, including depression and irritability, as well as loss of memory and hysteria, can develop. If the deficiency is severe, you can develop pellagra— dementia, dermatitis, and diarrhea.

- **Vitamin B-6** is required for production of several neurotransmitters, including serotonin. Deficiencies have been linked to emotional problems, depression, and tingling or numbness in hands and feet.

- **Vitamin B-12** (Cobalamin) is a component of myelin, that whitish tissue that covers your nerves. If you don't have enough of it, you can develop a disease called pernicious anemia, which can be fatal in extreme cases. A deficiency of B-12 can also cause emotional problems, neuritis, and lack of coordination in hands and legs. Some studies indicate there may be a connection between B-12 deficiency and Alzheimer type mental problems.

HOME
INSURANCE
POLICY

Your brain needs vitamins—and the B-complex is all important for Harmony's telephone system. But you should not increase any B-vitamin by itself—or you will throw Harmony off balance.

- **Antioxidants** - Another important group of nutrients for the nervous system is antioxidants. Free radicals increase the amount of damage to the brain when it suffers from oxygen deprivation (due to stroke, injury, disease, etc.). Research now indicates that antioxidants can help prevent this additional damage.

- **Electrolytes** conduct the electrical current so you can just imagine how significant they are to Harmony. Potassium, sodium and chloride salts are all electrolytes. Because it is so important, there should be about 250 grams of this mineral in your body, and the amounts of potassium and sodium must be in balance. When there is too much or too little of one or the other, Harmony can become unstable. Severe potassium deficiency can cause heart failure.

We've talked about brain food. Now, let's take a look at a few more wonderful features and benefits of your home's telephone system. For example, did you know that:

☎   Breathing is the only function of the autonomic nervous system that you can actually control. By intentionally altering the rate you breath, inhaling and exhaling, you can either stimulate or relax your nervous system. Rapid shallow breathing will speed lots of oxygen into your system. Intentional deep breathing can greatly relax you.

☎ Why does an object you are carrying feel heavier the longer you carry it? As muscles become tired, the nerves have to send stronger and stronger messages to the muscles to keep them working. Because your nerves also tell you that you are feeling something, the load you are *feeling* seems to be heavier because of the stronger messages.[52]

☎ If this is so, then why can you wear glasses on your face all day long but not continually *feel* them? Touch is our most sophisticated sense—it is all over our bodies. Harmony can actually use different pressure receptors to tell if the touch is gentle, hard, or vibrating. When the same touch continues for a period of time, such as wearing your glasses, the touch receptors send slower and slower announcements that the glasses are there.

☎ Did you know your awesome brain also oversees the development of your golf game or your ability to play tennis? You might wonder how this is possible.

When you learn to do something with your body, such as walking when you were a toddler, you program certain wiring patterns into your nervous system. By practicing the swing of that golf club or tennis racket, you are actually exercising your nervous system while your muscles are working. When you feel good about the swing, you transmit this information to central control. If you slice the golf ball or knock the tennis ball out of bounds, this data is also recorded. Over a period of time your brain is actually programmed to perform a certain technique.

The more you exercise the nervous system, the more efficient it will become. Research also seems to indicate that your nerves will live longer if they are exercised.

HOME
INSURANCE | *Reading is excellent exercise for your brain..* |
POLICY

☎   You have a left brain and a right brain and they are connected by a switchboard called the corpus callosum. The right side of the brain generally controls creative activities such as art and music, while the left side is used for analytical thinking like math.

☎   The limbic system (Latin word for *border*) is the central switchboard to your emotional feelings—love, hate, anger, fear, peace, joy, shame, and guilt to name a few. This switchboard connects brain structures that border the brain stem. Although you may actually *feel* emotions in your heart (i.e., a quickened heartbeat if you are frightened), they are actually the result of signals switched back and forth via the limbic system.

This overwhelming exchange of information between thoughts and feelings gives you the power of reasoning. A breakdown in this intricate switchboard can cause several disorders, including panic attacks.

Maintenance of your home's telephone system includes proper nutrition as well as natural therapies when something goes wrong. Herbs can be used to treat many ailments of the nervous system.

Dr. James Duke, a scientist at the USDA's Agricultural Research Service recommends the following herb teas for these ailments:

- Chamomile tea for soothing frazzled nerves
- Spearmint and peppermint for upset stomach
- Red raspberry tea to relax muscles
- Lemongrass or lavender for insomnia
- Rosehips for exposure to toxic environment

The telephone system in your home, with its 100 billion operators, carrying on 10,000 conversations each, is a very complex system—the most phenomenal one ever created. And it has about 75 trillion customers!

With such an awesome task, it is extremely important to maintain your nervous system, your communication network to Harmony.

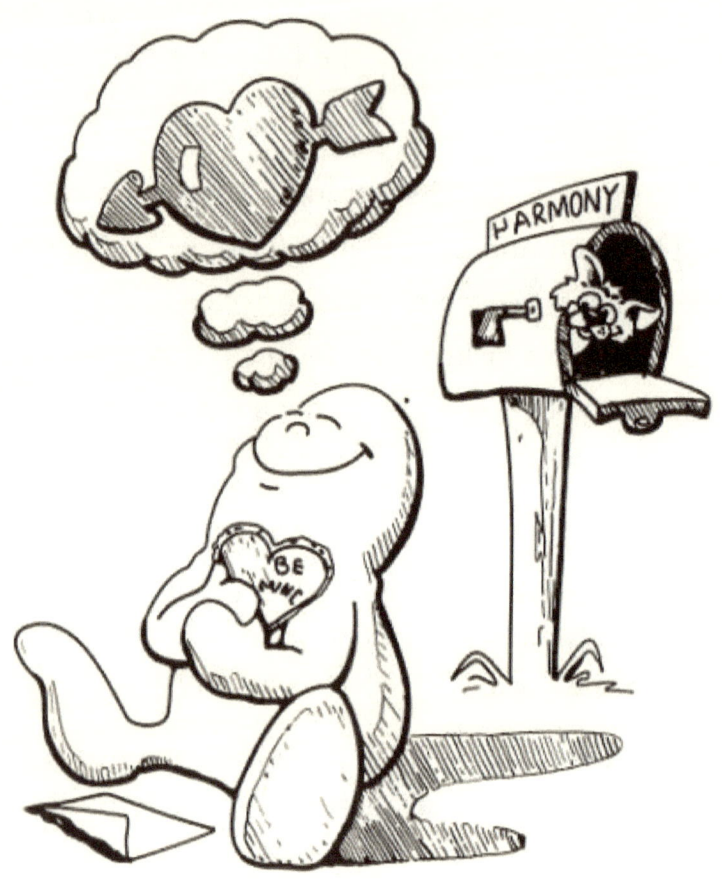

Food for Thought

Though reading and conversation may furnish us with many ideas, or men and things, yet it is our own meditation must form our judgment.

- Dr. I. Watts

Chapter 8

The Workout Room

Harmony in the Work Out Room is sadly lacking in many American homes. The word *exercise* conjures up visions of heavy duty weight lifters, marathon runners, or athletes who devote full time to sports. In fact, exercise is a method to make your body strong, healthy, and resistant to disease, so it will be a happy home for you for many, many years.

Shamefully, many of us give more attention to preventive maintenance of our cars than we do our own bodies.

Why is that?

The amazing creation that is your body requires oxygen in every cell in order to function properly. Exercise increases your respiration because your heart beats faster to take oxygen to the cells. This increases the flow of blood and adds more capillaries to the distribution system that carries vital nutrients to Harmony. Because more oxygen-rich nutrition is coming into the cell, and toxins are being removed just as quickly, Harmony is rejuvenated. When this happens seventy-five trillion times, your home becomes a very comfortable place in which to live; and it never wears out because it is constantly being repaired.

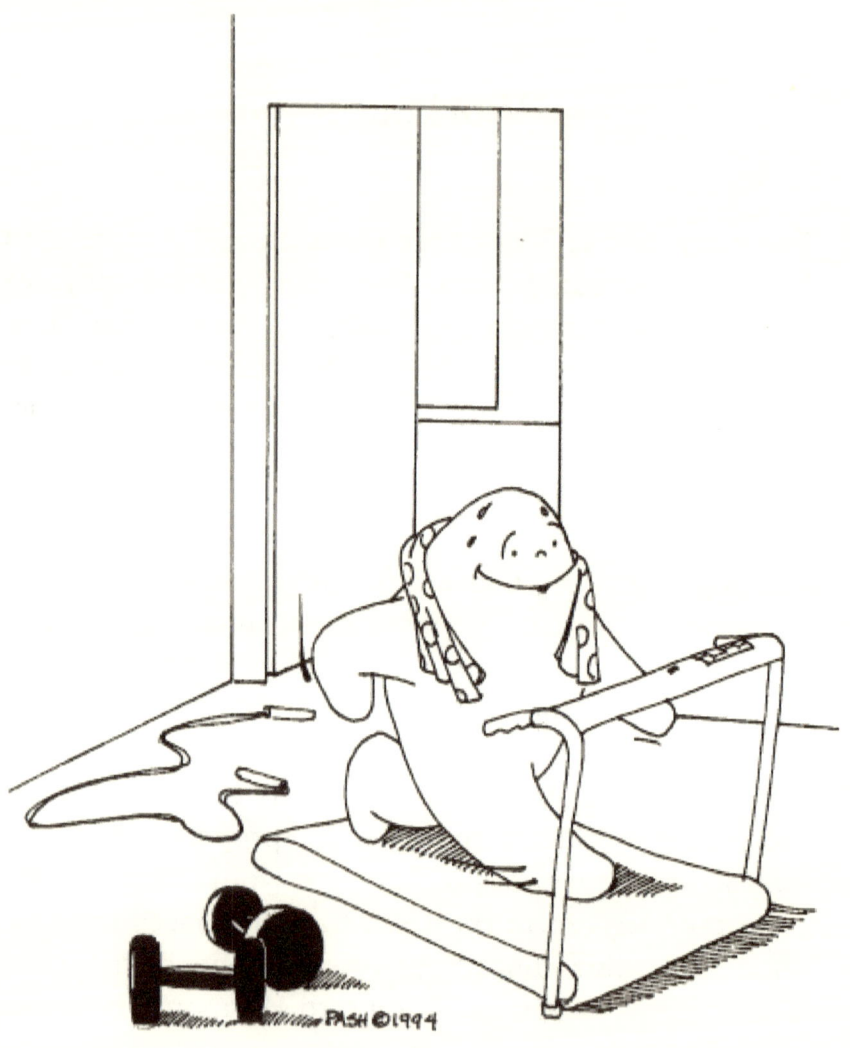

Do you have Harmony in your workout room?

HOME
INSURANCE
POLICY[53]

> *So many people 'rust out before they wear out,'*
> *observes one exercise expert, appropriately*
> *named Dr. Robert E. Wear, of the University of*
> *New Hampshire. He and other experts have*
> *found that a habit of exercise is about the closest*
> *thing we have to a fountain of youth.*
> — Nathaniel Lande

The human body was built for activity. When our prehistoric ancestors—homo sapiens—first appeared, activity and survival were synonymous. Woe be unto those who did not have powerful leg muscles to run from wild beasts, or sturdy arms for heaving spears. Living as children of nature, humans survived and thrived on the constant call to use their bodies.

HOME
INSURANCE
POLICY[54]

> *Many of the declines associated with aging are*
> *primarily the consequence of inactivity.*

With the evolution of societies, we grew further and further away from the lifestyle for which we were genetically and physiologically built. Our eating habits changed over the course of time and so did our level of physical activity. But our basic needs for natural food and natural exercise never changed. We have forgotten that we were designed to be physically active. Today, many of us say, *I don't have enough time to exercise.*

If you think you don't have time to exercise, ask yourself these questions:

- Do I have time to be sick?
- Do I have time it will take to recover?

We also complain that exercise is boring, not any fun, or simply not a priority. If these are your excuses, ask yourself this question:

- What is more important than taking care of me?

Nothing! Absolutely nothing is more important than taking care of yourself—and that includes exercise. So what are the advantages of regular exercise and why should you make it a part of your lifestyle?

Here is a brief list of just a few of the positive benefits you can reap from a physical activity program:

- Reduce body weight
- Increase muscle mass
- Improve bone strength
- Fight osteoporosis

Although you can't lose weight by exercise alone, toning and firming your muscles will help you look and feel better. Because muscles burn more calories than fat tissue, you will use more calories as muscle mass increases. Exercise can help reduce your appetite.

The skeletal system is strengthened by exercise. Built like a honeycomb (not solid as many imagine), bone cells must be constantly repaired or replaced just like other cells in the body. Exercise enhances this process, making bones stronger.

- Tone the heart muscle
- Increase lung capacity
- Improve circulation
- Increase tissue oxygen

The heart is the busiest muscle in your body. Like other muscles, the more it is used, the stronger it becomes. Exercise demands that the heart beat longer and stronger. This increased heart function calls for more oxygen, so your respiration increases, exercising the lungs and making them stronger. You now have extra oxygen in the blood stream, which is carried to all the body tissues, enhancing the performance of Harmony.

- Lower blood pressure
- Lower LDL (the lethal cholesterol)
- Raise HDL (the healthy cholesterol)

Regular aerobic exercise helps lower the blood pressure in mildly hypertensive people. After a period of time it can also lower LDL and triglycerides and raise your HDL.

- Improve digestive system
- Improve elimination
- Prevent hemorrhoids
- Reduce effects of varicose veins

Because exercise improves motility in the digestive tract, it helps reduce heartburn (an affliction of couch potatoes) and enhances the elimination process. If you are constipated, try taking a brisk walk for relief. People who sit a great deal are especially prone to hemorrhoids and need exercise to improve circulation. The faster the heart is pumping, the faster blood is circulated, eliminating *pooling* and reducing hemorrhoids. The same is true for varicose veins. Get your heart pumping and keep that blood circulating!

- Decrease tension and stress

In response to stress, the adrenal glands release the stimulant adrenalin. To balance the effects of stress on your body, the brain manufactures serotonin and norepinephrine (neurotransmitters). When these neurotransmitters are in short supply, and you are stressed, you are more prone to depression. Because exercise increases the supply of these neurotransmitters, you are guarding yourself from the effects of stress with your own built in protection.[55]

- Enhance the immune system
- Inhibit cancer growth[56]
- Lower risk for disease

Exercise can help you generate white blood cells, the body's army that fights invaders. Because exercise also raises your body temperature slightly, the white blood cells produce a protein called pyrogen. This protein reinforces the work of the lymphocytes. In addition, "high temperatures have also been shown to kill cancer cells."[57] When the immune system works properly, you lower the risk for disease.

- Help control diabetes

By increasing metabolism, and subsequent utilization of glucose, exercise can reduce the need for insulin.

- Combat chronic fatigue syndrome

This disease is a result of poor immunity and the condition is aggravated by stress. Exercise improves the immune system and helps alleviate stress, which reduces the symptoms of this disorder.

- Lengthen life

When you are healthy, your body can resist deadly afflictions such as heart disease and cancer. When you are free of disease, you can live a long and productive life in a state of wellness.

HOME
INSURANCE
POLICY

> *Exercise is a vital ingredient in the recipe for wellness.*

With all these benefits why would you choose not to exercise?

We know that prevention is the most economical health care you can buy. Regular exercise is a large portion of any prevention program. Spending minutes a day to exercise can just possibly save you many, many hours of illness and recuperation time. Because of Harmony's tremendous ability to repair itself when it has the right tools, it is never too late for you to start a regular workout program and reap the rewards of wellness.

HOME	*Cancer statistics will continue to climb*
INSURANCE	*as long as the formula for our lifestyle*
POLICY	*= obesity + no exercise + junk food.*

So now you've decided to start exercising, you need to know where to begin. First, remember that any lifestyle change should be done carefully over a period of time. You can't turn all those 75 trillion sedentary couch potato cells into physically fit athletes overnight.

Then:

1. **Get a check-up** that includes a medical history and electrocardiogram (ECG) to be sure your heart can handle increased activity.

2. **Make a plan**. What do you want to achieve? Do you need to lose weight, or just tone up? Do you want to build muscle confirmation like Charles Atlas or be a lean runner? Do you want to take up some sport you enjoyed in your youth?

3. Start by doing a few simple things. Leave your car on the distant side of the parking lot, climb stairs instead of riding elevators, take a walk every day.

4. Make time for you! Set aside time for your own individualized program. Sign up for that dancing class or join a health club. Buy good running shoes, or outfit yourself for bicycling.

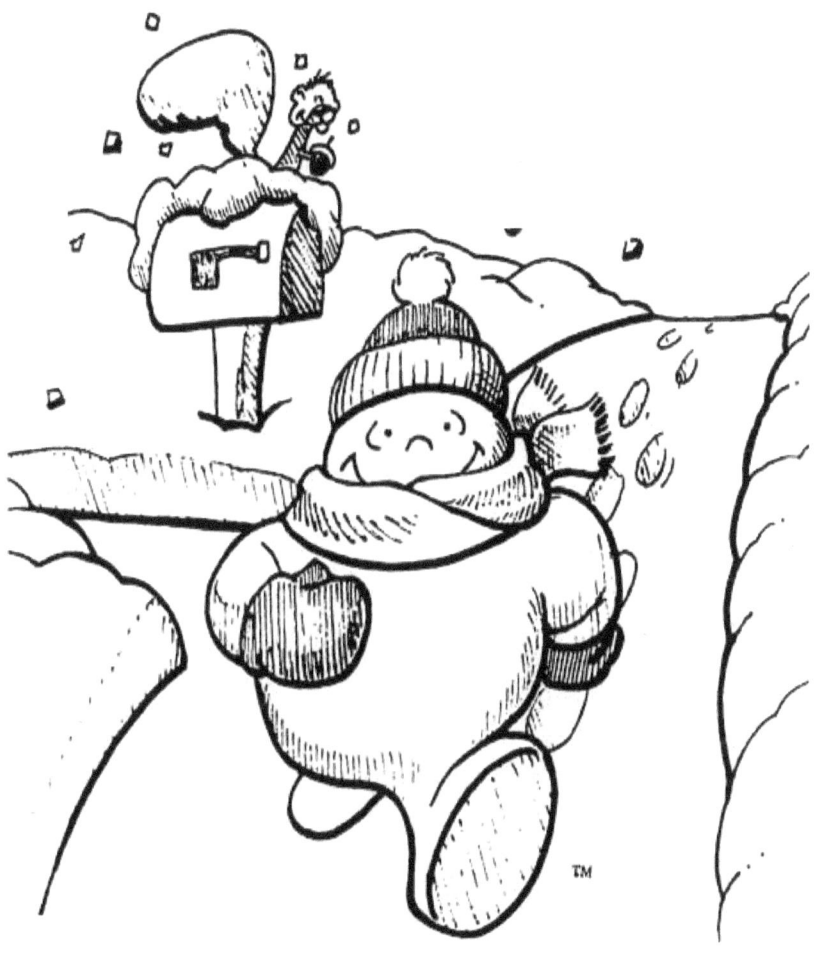

Walking can be very good for you!

5. Increase your activity level to your desired goal. Ideally, you should exercise so that your heart beat is between 70 and 80 percent of the maximum for your age. (See appendix.)

6. Be realistic. If something hurts, stop. If you experience chest pain, rapid heartbeat, shortness of breath, upset stomach, etc., call your doctor immediately.

7. Stick to it. Given time, your body has incredible powers of rejuvenation and renewal, so don't expect to have a new body in just a few days. As your stamina, health, and mental attitude change, you'll wonder why it took you so long to exercise your way into the state of wellness.

HOME INSURANCE POLICY	*Why don't health insurance companies "rate" their policy holders the way car insurers do —the more the risk the higher the cost?*

Now that we've looked at the benefits of exercise, do you know how to get started?

Do you know which kind of exercise you want to do?

Warm-up is the first rule of exercising. Why? Because it will loosen up those muscles, joints, tendons and ligaments. This will reduce chances of injury from over-exertion. By giving a boost to your respiration, it also increases your circulation.

Cardio-vascular, circulatory-respiratory, and aerobic are three names given to exercises that all work on your heart, lungs and circulation. This type of exercise includes walking, jogging, bicycling, rope jumping, and swimming. Tennis and soccer are two of the many competitive sports that will give you a good cardio-vascular workout.

Strength and endurance, body building and weight training are names given to repetitive exercises that work on specific areas of the body. These include activities like sit-ups, deep knee bends, push-ups, leg raises, arm circles, and working with weights.

Your body was created for health and happiness and activity is a key to the state of wellness. A regular exercise program will enhance your outlook on life and your overall appearance. When you sow exercise in your lifestyle, you'll reap the rewards of health.

People seldom improve when they have no other model but themselves to copy.
> - Goldsmith

...success is to be measured not so much by the position that one has reached in life as by the obstacles which he has overcome while trying to succeed.
> - Booker T. Washington

CHAPTER 9

The Medicine Cabinet

When you cut your finger or get the sniffles, chances are you go to the medicine cabinet and search its contents for something that will give you relief. If you want to live in a state of wellness, you will provide Harmony with natural healing herbs and remedies for the day to day discomforts of colds, allergies, aches and pains.

Drugs—those chemical concoctions manufactured by the pharmaceutical giants—do not heal. Drugs treat symptoms only! Your splendid body heals itself when provided the necessary tools for the job.

But finding the right tools can be an awesome task! Even natural therapies can have numerous treatments for specific disorders.

- How do you know which one to choose?
- If you decide on vitamin or mineral therapies, do you know how much you should take?
- Will the high increase in one supplement create a deficiency in another?

- There are so many health practitioners, how do you choose one?
- What about alternative or holistic therapies?
- What are they and how do they work?
- Should you try them?
- Are they safe?

And the most important question of all:

- How do you restore balance in the body when Harmony is in chaos?

So many questions—who has the right answers? The first thing to remember is this:

No one practitioner has all the right answers, and no one modality is right all the time.

If there was only one right way to treat illness and restore health, we would not have such a wide range of choices. The fact is, there are many therapies available to us today because they each have merits. They also have detractors.

| HOME INSURANCE POLICY | *The doctor of the future will give no medicine but will interest his patients in the care of the human frame, in diet, and in the cause and prevention of disease.*   - Thomas A. Edison |

Find the combination that works for you. You are a unique person. You should seek the therapist and treatments that are right for you and you alone.

HOME INSURANCE POLICY[58]	*A study published in the* New England Journal of Medicine *last year showed that one in three Americans now uses alternative healers.* - Jan Goodwin

The second thing to remember is this: The person who practices medicine on themselves may have a short-lived career. Treating yourself can be dangerous!

The key to the state of wellness will belong to the person who knows that there are many modalities available today and is willing to give complementary or alternative therapies an opportunity to work for them.

If you are sick and tired of being sick and tired maybe it's time to learn about some of the many paths you can take to wellness.

So what are these alternative modalities and therapies that can lead you to wellness?

We'll list the various practices first and then we'll discuss some of the alternative therapies.

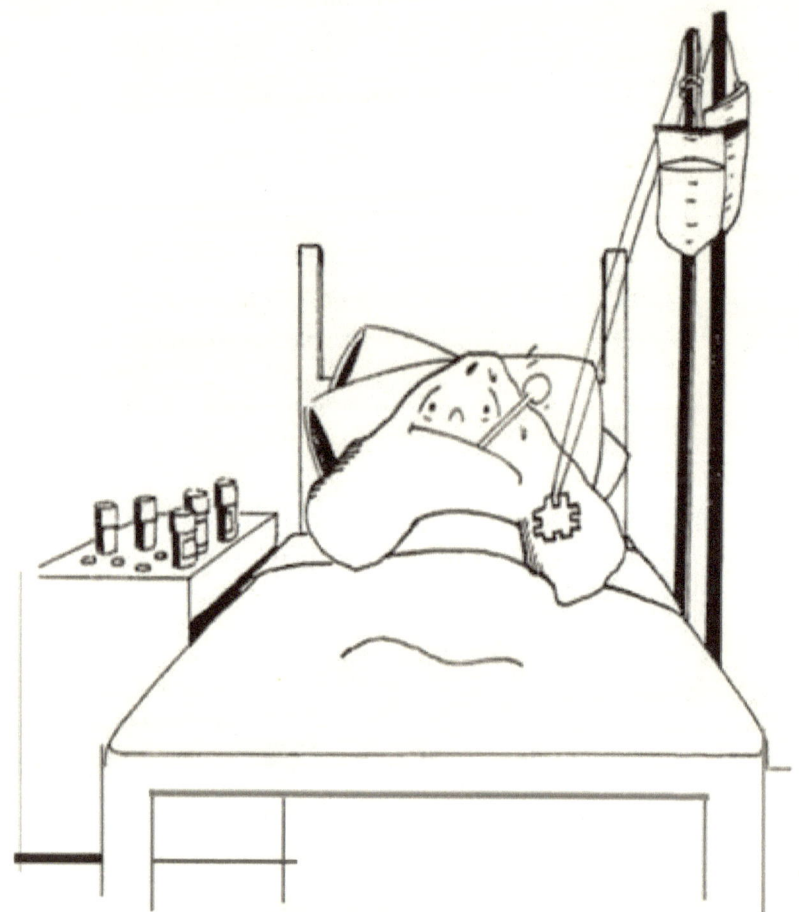

Harmony in chaos.

Acupuncture has been used for thousands of years. It is an ancient Chinese method of healing that uses needles to realign the energy that flows through the body. By inserting very fine needles at various meridian points, the energy that flows to specific organs can be manipulated. Acupuncture is widely accepted throughout the United States and is effective in the treatment of chronic pain.

> *[acupuncture] reduces pain and anxiety, stabilizes blood-sugar and cholesterol levels, and improves sleep and body functioning—all of which help the body fight back.*
>
> - Dr. Semmler de la Torre

Allopathic Medicine is a method of treating disease by alleviating the symptoms. Medical doctors practice allopathy and generally consider themselves to be the traditional healers. But allopathic medicine is a relative new-comer to the world of medical arts, and allopathic drugs have only been around since the early 1900's.

Medical doctors may claim that alternative therapies work because the patient thought they would work. Who is to say that the same is not true of allopathic medicine—that the patients of medical doctors recover from illness simply because they think they will, and not because the doctor actually did anything that *cured* the patient. When it comes to medications, how do we know that all drugs, regardless of their source, are not having a placebo effect?

Eighteen years ago the nationally circulated *USA Today* said in the cover story on July 27, 1994, that "Education on medications is 'terrible'" and went on to say that drugs are mis-prescribed by doctors to one-fourth of America's elderly citizens.[60]

Sadly, in all these years, we have done little to nothing to improve this situation.   In 2011, there were 179,855 serious or fatal Adverse Drug Reactions (ADRs).[61]

HOME
INSURANCE
POLICY[62]

> *Medical schools and conferences are supported or sponsored by drug manufacturers, who are not interested in promoting nutritional therapies.*
> - Zoltan P. Rona, M.D., M.Sc.

Chiropractors believe that misalignment of nerve pathways causes disease and manipulation of the spine, or other areas of the body, relieves the stress that caused the illness. It is particularly useful in the treatment of back and joint pain associated with muscle spasms.

Holistic doctors look at the whole person to diagnose and treat disease rather than depending upon one system or part. They believe that the mind, body, and spirit must all be employed if the patient is to become well. Many holistic practitioners employ a variety of modalities that may include acupuncture, chiropractic, homeopathy, aromatherapy, allopathy, iridology, herbal therapies, and vitamin/mineral supplementation.

Homeopathy treats *like with like*. For instance, a person with insomnia might be treated with a minuscule portion of caffeine that alters the flow of the life force in the body, resulting in a peaceful sleep. It is especially effective in the treatment of chronic problems such as allergies, arthritis and hypertension.

Because homeopathy relies heavily on the body to heal itself over a period of time, it should never be used in the case of medical emergency or serious infection.

Homeopathy, as it is practiced today, has been used more than 200 years, although the basis for this ancient healing art has been known for thousands of years. Writing in *Health Counselor* newsletter Frances FitzGerald says that "...as the 20th century comes to a close, there is an increasing dissatisfaction over mainstream medicine's expense, questionable effectiveness, and sometimes dangerous side effects ."[63]

She goes on to say that "many physicians and patients agree that homeopathy, a natural healing science, deserves a closer look."[64]

This field of medical science holds much promise for non-invasive treatment of numerous medical maladies in the future. And homeopathy is now being used by holistic veterinarians with astounding success.[65] Here in the year 2012, there is continued dissatisfaction in health care, yet homeopathy is still not a mainstream modality.

Why?

Iridologists diagnose disease and imminent illness by studying the iris of the eye. Like acupuncture or chiropractic, meridian points of the body are reflected in the iris and study of the texture and structure of the iris can lead to non-invasive diagnosis. Iridology is a diagnostic tool used by many health practitioners, including medical doctors.

Kinesiology employs the neuro-muscular system for diagnosis and treatment. It is sometimes called A.K., or applied kinesiology.

Naturopaths use natural therapies that enable the body to heal without invasive procedures. They believe that disease is caused by lack of proper maintenance of the body allowing the immune system to be overtaken by poor lifestyle factors such as stress and improper nutrition.

Osteopathy is based on the theory that a sound body depends upon the health and maintenance of the body's structures.

Although osteopaths may use their hands-on approach to diagnose disease and manipulate body structures to treat problems, many today conduct their practices along the lines of allopathic medical doctors by prescribing drugs and using x-rays. There are also osteopathic specialist and surgeons such as urologists and orthopedists.

HOME
INSURANCE
POLICY

> *When you've finished changing, you're finished.*
> - Benjamin Franklin

With all these choices, how do you choose a reliable health practitioner?

First:
- Get references from friends or family members; advertisements can be misleading or even false.

- Ask your reference how they were helped.

- Was the therapy beneficial?

- Was it reasonably priced?

- Was the office staff competent and professional?

Second:
- Check out the doctor's credentials.

- What do all those initials after their name mean?

- Did they receive a formal education?

- What health associations have admitted them as members?

Third:
- Watch out for exorbitant claims. Do they claim to have secret knowledge or a cure-all pill?

- If so, you'll want to avoid them.

The human mind is the most powerful healing resource in the world. You can be as sick or as well as you think you are.

Now let's take a look at some of the many complementary, alternative, or integrative therapies that are available:

Aromatherapy uses fragrances from plants, flowers, and fruits for relaxation and pain relief from disorders such as headaches, arthritis, and nasal congestion. Various aromatic oils are used to treat certain maladies but should not be taken internally. Use them only by inhalation under the supervision of a licensed practitioner or by rubbing diluted oils into the skin.

Biofeedback monitors skin temperature, muscle tension, and other body processes by using sensors that send data to a machine. The machine continually produces a graph of the patient's responses and by watching the readings patients learn to control their thoughts and movements. Biofeedback is effective in pain control as well as other disorders such as hypertension, psychological phobias, and anxiety.

Chelation Therapy removes calcium from the arteries as well as heavy metal toxics such as mercury and lead. The patient receives an intravenous solution of vitamins, minerals, and EDTA (a synthetic amino acid called ethylene diamine tera-acetic acid), which extracts the harmful chemicals from the circulatory system and eliminates them through the kidneys.

EDTA was developed in Germany in 1935, as an alternative to citric acid and has been used as a preservative in hundreds of products. Starting in the 1950's many research papers by distinguished scientists and articles in medical journals demonstrated the effective use of chelation therapy in the treatment of atherosclerosis, arteriosclerosis, circulation disorders, and toxic metal poisoning. Among the side benefits are improvements in arthritis and diabetes, improved stamina, and better memory.

Chelation therapy can lower the need for certain medicines that may create toxicity in the body. Combined with exercise, vitamin-mineral supplements and diet, it is a proven treatment for coronary artery disease and other circulatory problems.

Colonics cleanses the bowels. Many health practitioners believe that all disease originates in the colon and thus it should be cleaned regularly. This practice may be good for some people but totally unnecessary, or even harmful to others. If you think it would be beneficial, check out some of the non-invasive methods for maintaining bowel health, such as herbal colon cleansers.

Always re-flora the system (with a good pro-biotic that is taken orally) after a cleansing to restore the good bacteria necessary for proper assimilation and elimination.

Fasting helps Harmony eliminate toxic accumulations. During a fast the body burns damaged or diseased parts which are then expelled through the skin, lungs, kidneys or colon. There are many types of cleansing and detoxifying fasts, which can last from one to ten days. Many people who fast regularly report they are not only physically healthier, but also enjoy a heightened awareness and more positive outlook on life.

If you are interested in a fasting program, it is probably better to start with a one-day juice fast and work up to a longer regimen. Be sure to follow the guidelines of a health professional any time you fast.

Hair Analysis measures the amount of minerals and heavy toxic metals in the body. For accuracy, the hair is taken from the back of the head, as close to the scull as possible. Some labs can compensate for the effects of dyes or shampoos on the hair itself. Others may not be so reliable. Used in combination with blood tests and urinalysis, hair analysis can be a valuable method of determining the overall condition of Harmony.

Hypnosis uses the mind to overcome fears or anxieties as well as treating pain and other therapeutic applications, such as sleep disorders, overeating, and smoking and other addictive disorders. If you have a specific medical complaint, or do not feel well, you should have a comprehensive evaluation before undergoing hypnosis.

Massage Therapy was recommended in a Chinese book 2700 B.C. and has been around ever since. There are several styles of massage therapy; the Swedish is most common in this country. The Eastern style attempts to balance energy paths, while Western works on muscles and connective tissue. Massage induces relaxation and helps improve mobility.

Reflexology is a therapy that uses massage and pressure on the hands and/or feet to treat various organs. Based on principles similar to acupuncture or iridology, it is sometimes called zone therapy.

Therapeutic Touch is based on two ancient healing doctrines: Laying-on-of-hands and energy flow. By receiving energy from the healer's hands, the patient's hemoglobin levels can be raised, restoring their vitality.

HOME
INSURANCE
POLICY

> *...you will discover that your health, happiness, and the future of life on earth are rarely so much in your own hands as when you sit down to eat.*
> - John Robbins

Taking care of the human body, the incomparable creation, is an art as old as mankind. There are many, many options for health treatments that have been around for thousands of years, and that fact alone would give them some credibility. But don't wait until you have a health crisis to seek out advice and treatments from complementary/alternative therapies or practitioners. These modalities are generally based on the theory that the human body can mend itself, given the proper tools and time. In the event of an emergency, you should seek the immediate assistance of a medical doctor.

Now that we have reviewed some of the therapies that are available today, let's take a look at some of the natural products that Harmony might want you to keep in the medicine cabinet. (For a more extensive list of herbs see Appendix.)

Aloe vera

—has been used for more than 4000 years to treat hundreds of ailments. The fact that it is mentioned in the Bible five times would seem to add credibility to its healing properties. Although frequently referred to as a "natural drug," aloe vera is actually a nutrient that improves the body's immune system. With an improved immune system, the body can more effectively fight diseases—even deadly ones like cancer and AIDS.

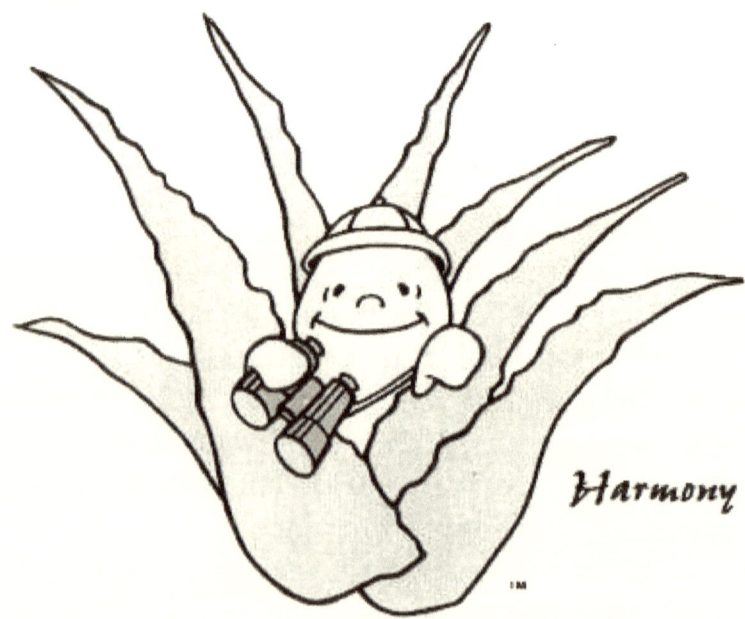

Harmony

Unfortunately, this valuable nutrient, probably the greatest healing agent in the history of the world, has never been approved by the Federal Drug Administration for therapeutic medical applications in the United States.

Why?

Because an FDA approval costs anywhere from $100 to $300 million dollars—and aloe vera cannot be patented since it is a plant.[66] Without the protection of a patent, which would generate many millions (perhaps billions) of dollars of revenue for the patent holder, no one will go through the expensive FDA approval process.

Without any sort of control over the manufacture and distribution of this incredible healing substance, there are numerous suppliers in the United States who sell the product in much less than therapeutic formulas. These watered down aloe vera products have no efficacy, and yet sell for high prices.

If you want to try aloe vera, purchase a whole leaf cold processed formulation. And be sure you take the product daily. Like other herbal remedies, it takes time to improve the body's immune system so that Harmony can be restored.

HOME INSURANCE POLICY	*Everything you need in your medicine cabinet can be found in nature.*

Chromium enhances the energy level and keeps it stable throughout the day by improving the metabolism of glucose. For this reason people with diabetes and hypoglycemia find that it is an important companion for Harmony.

The typical American diet may have only 25 micrograms of this essential trace mineral yet the average person needs 400 to 1000 mcg. a day. That's quite a deficiency!

The minimum requirement for wellness is greatly increased if you eat a lot of refined sugar or exercise— since your body needs chromium to handle both these functions.

Numerous studies on chromium polynicotinate indicate that it not only helps the body burn fat, it also enhances muscle formation, reduces cholesterol, and balances insulin. It can be an important part of your medicine cabinet supplies if you have diabetes or need to lose weight.

HOME INSURANCE POLICY	*For the earth which drinks in the rain that often comes upon it, and bears herbs useful for those by whom it is cultivated, receives blessings from God.* - Hebrews 6:7

Here are a few more healthy hints for Harmony's medicine cabinet:

Colds - Does your medicine cabinet contain any of the over-the-counter cold remedies? If so, you ought to think about throwing them away.

Why is that?

Cold symptoms—runny nose, watery eyes, chest congestion, and coughing—are really the body's attempt to fight off an assaulting cold virus. When one of the more than 200 cold viruses invades Harmony, the cells fight back with white blood cells. To help your army identify the enemy, proteins floating in the blood stream surround the enemy and cover them. That's when you notice the sore throat, start sneezing, and hang on to the Kleenex box so you can blow away all those nasty germs.

What happens if you inhibit this process? Have you ever had one cold right after another? Chances are you never gave Harmony a chance to completely wipe out the enemy.

What should you do when you have a cold?

Many have found that increasing Vitamin C helps. Also, drink more fluids, especially fresh fruit juices, to help flood the enemy out of your home.

(Personally, I eat the white pulp between the fruit and the outer skin of a grapefruit, and I also chew the seeds thoroughly. I have found this approach to be very effective and never have a cold more than three days.)

Rest may be necessary, especially if you have a fever. Natural therapies such as these can help alleviate symptoms without inhibiting the healing process. Remember, when you have a cold, Harmony is at war. If you inhibit the process, you'll surely be imprisoning some of the enemy. Why in the world would you want to do that?

HOME INSURANCE POLICY	*The Lord created medicines from the earth, and a sensible man will not disparage them.* - Ecclesiastes 38:4.

Cuts and Abrasions - Do you know what the best topical antibiotic is? Strange as it may seem, you probably won't find a more effective treatment than plain old refined table sugar for killing those bacteria on a minor cut or abrasion. Not only does the sugar take care of the bad guys already on the site, it also inhibits the growth of more.

Colloidal Silver is a natural antibiotic that kills more than 650 kinds of single-cell bacteria, so it can effectively treat many ailments. It has been used since the late 1800s, and was grandfathered in as an approved antibiotic when the FDA was established in 1906 with the passage of the Pure Food and Drugs Act.

A good suspension will be 5 parts per million. It should always be taken with a plastic spoon, since metal can attract the silver particles and thus reduce its effectiveness. Colloidal silver can be used on open wounds as well as in the eyes and ears. There are documented cases of it being used successfully to treat life-threatening diseases such as hepatitis and gangrene.

A few drops of colloidal silver sniffed in the nose can be very effective for treating sinus infections, and if you have a burn, you'll find it to be not only soothing, but immensely therapeutic as well.

Juicing has many therapeutic applications. It is an effective way of getting mammoth portions of nutrition into your body without a lot of bulk. Although the process may leave a mess to clean, the benefits far outweigh the inconvenience. With juicing you can consume the nutrients from a pound of carrots in glass!

Since most poor health is a result of improper nutrition, quickly providing your cells with the vital nutrients they need can produce miraculous results in Harmony. Only fifteen minutes after drinking fresh prepared vegetable or fruit juices on an empty stomach, you are sending life-restoring vitamins and minerals, enzymes, amino acids and proteins to your 75 trillion cells.

Results of juicing have been documented for many years, and people new to juicing add to the large school of proponents. Testimonies continue to affirm the healing powers of fresh, raw vegetable juices as people recover from arthritic diseases, circulatory and respiratory problems, digestion and elimination ailments, nervous conditions, and weight disorders—either overweight from excessive eating or underweight from inability to eat at all.

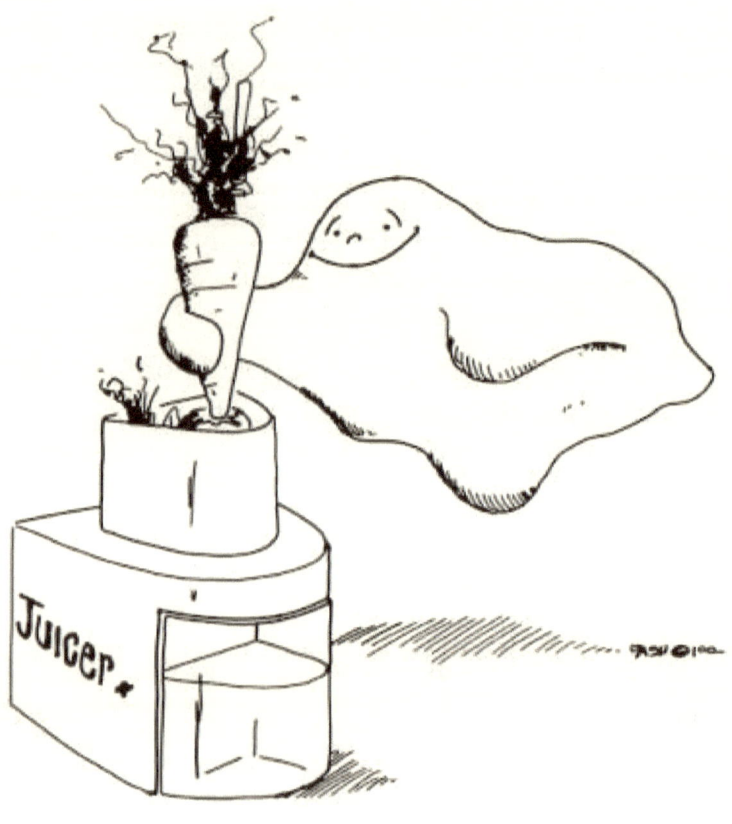

Why is juicing so effective for so many ailments?

The answer lies in organic sodium, which is needed so the body can use calcium. If the calcium is not in the proper solution it gets stuck in various places. If it's in the joints, you have arthritis; in the kidney, kidney stones; in the gall bladder, gall stones; in the arteries, arteriosclerosis. High concentrations of organic sodium in the juice of celery and cucumbers quickly restores Harmony's balance and takes calcium where it belongs.

HOME
INSURANCE
POLICY[67]

The U.S. Public Health Service is spending $13 million this year on studies of alternative treatments, including several on herbs and plant compounds.   -Leslie Miller

The list of natural remedies is endless, and countless books have been written about them. Now that you are aware of a few perhaps you'll give them a try. We know that the cures for all our ailments can be found in nature. If you are out of balance, and seem to be losing Harmony, check out the contents of nature's medicine cabinet.

Food for Thought

For there exist in our possession
hidden treasures in the field,
wheat and barley and oil and honey.
                    - Jeremiah 41:8

CHAPTER 10

The Home Security System

How secure is your home?
Do you have burglar bars on the windows to keep the bad guys out?

Or do you have a monitored alarm system that automatically calls the police? Perhaps you just have a barking dog. Maybe you feel safe and don't worry about burglars breaking into your home.

As a child you may have had the happy experience of growing up in a secure community—and you never even had to lock the doors. Do you remember the annual search for the house key before leaving on vacation so the house could be locked during the week-long absence?

If you have such memories, chances are you grew up in a place where the air was clean and pure, the food was always fresh and wholesome, and living in wellness was the norm.

Today's lifestyle is quite different. We live in high density communities where air pollution is common, processed foods are routine, and home security systems are a requirement.

How secure is your body's home—the incredible creation in which you live?

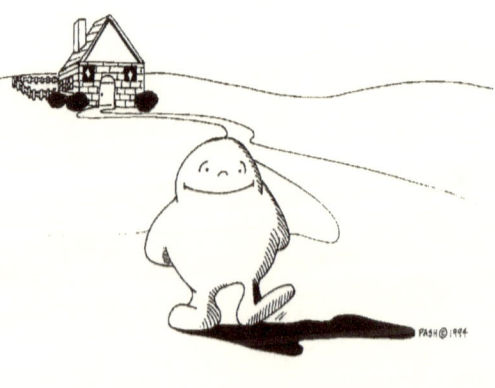

Do you take time each day to set the alarm system and lock the doors?

Or do you go on that once-a-year search for home security by subjecting yourself to the rigors of an annual physical examination at your doctor's office?

Perhaps you have never even thought about securing your body with wellness each and every day. Why?

Would you leave the doors on your house unlocked if a band of burglars was marauding your neighborhood on a regular basis?

Wouldn't you be courting disaster if you didn't take some simple precautions to protect your house?

Don't you think you should protect your body, too?

Maybe you feel that your home/body is perfectly safe. Or maybe the thought of securing your home is a scary idea to you because if you admit that you need to take precautions you're giving in to your fear of disease.

That is nonsense.

The wise and prudent person will lock their house and sleep soundly at night knowing that they are safe from the prowling band of thieves. They will be comfortable and secure.

Don't you think you owe the same care to your wonderful body?

If you still think the idea of a home security system is unnecessary, perhaps you should become familiar with some of these statistics in the United States:

- Heart disease is the number one killer in this country;

- Cancer is the second most common cause of death;

- By the year 2020, 1 person in 19 will have cancer[68];

- Despite various new therapies, there has been no significant improvement in cancer treatment;

- So few people die of natural causes there are no statistics.

Dr. Charles B. Simone, a leading oncologist, says in his book *Cancer & Nutrition*, "...nutrition, lifestyle, and the environment are the most common risk factors for cancer" and that these factors account for 80-90 percent of all cancers. That is a powerful statement, yet Dr. Simone has all the facts and figures to substantiate his assertions.[69]

HOME
INSURANCE
POLICY

> *You have the right to know the risks.*
> *It is your responsibility to reduce them.*

Do you know which organs of the body are most commonly attacked by cancer?

According to Dr. Simone, other than the skin, it is the lungs, the breasts, the colon, and the rectum.

You might want to believe that lifestyle has nothing to do with cancer, or causing cancer. The facts speak for themselves and here are just a few. A complete list would be endless.

- Women who eat high fat diets are much more likely to develop breast cancer. (Men also develop breast cancer.)

- Smoking is directly linked to lung cancer. Air pollution may also be a risk factor for this type of cancer.

- There are carcinogens in our drinking water. Since 1940, over 70,000 chemicals have been added to our lifestyle.

- The immune system was designed to protect your body. Allergies, antibiotics, refined carbohydrates and excessive consumption of animal fats all depress the immune system.[70]

Free radicals have come to the forefront of health news in the last decade or so, and we've all been told to take anti-oxidants to combat them. This is excellent advice. However, do you really understand what this scientific gibberish means?

What do free radicals do to your body anyway?

Free radicals are the atomic by-product of the continual chemical reactions that take place in our bodies. They are called *radicals* because they are just that—they are like angry, fanatic revolutionaries roaming around the countryside stirring up trouble.

Why are they so angry?

To answer this question you need to understand atoms. Each atom has a nucleus, which is surrounded by electrons, sort of like the leader of a gang surrounded by the members of the gang. They all hang out together.

The leader is very powerful and carries a positive charge. The gang members each have a small negative charge, but all together their power is equal to the leader's clout. Everyone in the gang is happy as long as the power of their organization is stable at zero—the power of all the negatives is equal to all the power of the positives.

HOME
INSURANCE
POLICY[71]

Now, scientists believe they are finally standing before cancer's last stronghold, the cell itself.
Shannon Brownlee
U.S. News & World Report

In a split-fraction of a second an outlaw from another gang comes over to this happy little band of thieves and throws out one of their member electrons and takes its place in the gang. (The outlaw can be from any sort of gang: alcohol, polyunsaturated fats, radiation, smog, tobacco, or any other group that is foreign to the body.)

The evicted electron is really mad. It no longer has a gang to hang out with; so, it goes on a rampage and finds another atom gang and jumps into it.

Now this gang is thrown into a wild rage because of all the new energy it has accumulated. With the addition of the evicted electron, the gang becomes a free radical and goes on a shooting spree to use up all its out-of-balance energy. During the shooting spree it does a lot of damage to the surrounding countryside.

The countryside is all the tissues in your body—your precious home. Now the air around your home is full of oxygen, right? Harmony cannot survive without oxygen.

When these marauding gangs invade an oxygen atom, and turn it into a free radical, it is very dangerous. It invades Harmony's home and revolutionizes the cell, so it no longer works the way it should. This is the start of many diseases such as cancer, emphysema, heart disease, atherosclerosis, immune system disorders, rheumatoid arthritis, cataracts, dementia, kidney and gastrointestinal diseases, and aging.

That's right. Free radicals cause aging!

But there is a way to keep these wild gang members under control. If you hire the posse, they can round up all the bad guys and send them to jail where they will be hung.

What sort of posse can rescue you?

They are called the ACES: Vitamins A, C, E, and the mineral selenium. And they are the very best posse you will ever know.

Together they are known as anti-oxidants because they stop the wild oxygen free radicals from damaging (oxidizing) your body. In order to work, though, you must take enough to be effective.

The Vitamin E members of the posse actually surround the polyunsaturated fat molecules and fight over the free radicals. If you have more Vitamin E posse members than polyunsaturated fat molecules, Vitamin E will win. And so will you! Without enough Vitamin E, the fat molecules will capture the free radicals and you'll be stuck will all those outlaws in your cells.

| HOME INSURANCE POLICY | *Free radicals are dangerous.* *Did you install a security system* *to maintain Harmony in your home?* |

CHAPTER 11

A Trip to the Playground

The typical American diet includes generous servings of coffee, colas and ice cream—caffeine and sugar laden treats that taste good to the palate. We each eat 150 pounds of sugar a year[72] which is up 30 pounds just since 1995! Forty-three million of us are addicted to nicotine[73] and twelve million[74] of us are alcoholics.

No one knows how many people have a caffeine dependence, although one survey in Vermont indicated that 3% of caffeine users had a *severe* dependence while 14% has a *moderate* dependence.[75]

Over a period of time these substances all take a toll on Harmony—they create chaos in your 75 trillion cells. Sugar, caffeine, and nicotine are foreign substances to the human body. Your cells were not created to process them. They have no nutritional value, and yet we eat, drink and smoke them for the pleasurable effects we think they produce. We eat sugar for energy, drink caffeine to wake up, and smoke nicotine to calm down.

We consume them for one reason, but in the long run they all have the opposite effect on your body. They are playing games on you!! When you coddle your cravings for caffeine, colas, and *coffin nails* you are courting disaster—you are taking a very dangerous trip to the playground.

HOME INSURANCE POLICY	*Caffeine, sugar, and nicotine play havoc with Harmony*

Are these substances really so bad? What do they do to you anyway?

If they are unhealthy, why are they so readily available? To answer these questions, let's take a look at their historical and economic backgrounds.

The religious books of wisdom, including the Torah, the New Testament, and the Koran, all record information about the diets of our ancient ancestors—and what they could or could not eat. Sugar was never mentioned in any of these texts. Many of the people recorded in these books lived very long, long lives.

There is historical evidence that the ancient Greeks and Romans enjoyed the sweetness of cane and a writer in the time of Nero is credited with naming the sweet substance *saccharum.* Around 600 A.D. the University of Djondisapour in Persia developed a process that turned the natural sugar in the cane plant into a solid form that would not ferment and the sugar industry was born.[76]

HOME
INSURANCE
POLICY

> *Sugar was not served in the Garden of Eden.*

With the rise of Islam, the use of sugar became widespread and even the crusaders developed a taste for Saracens.[77]   In 1306, an appeal was sent to Pope Clement V outlining a plan to renew the Crusades, overthrow the Sultan, and take over the sugar fields in Cyprus, Malta, and Sicily. These sugar fields produced huge incomes and taxes.

With the race for production of sugar, and the money it generated, the Portuguese developed plantations in Valencia and Granada. Since they needed workers, Africans were kidnapped and shipped to the Iberian peninsula. This gave rise to hundreds of years of devastating slavery—all for the sake of sugar and money!

HOME
INSURANCE
POLICY

> *Don't you be a slave to sugar.*

As sugar production spread throughout Europee, great wealth was generated for the royalty, along with new sugar related diseases. When the British took over the West Indies, and the lucrative sugar plantations, they started a new business with fermented sugar—rum.

Rum also turned into a pot of gold. It was sold to American Indians in exchange for furs. In Europe, these furs were sold for fortunes.

HOME INSURANCE POLICY	*Confinement of the insane began in the 1600's— along with the increase in consumption of sugar.*

In 1573, a journal written by German botanist Leonhard Rauwolf, who was traveling in Libya and Tripoli, reported that the Turks and Moors had become gluttonous on sugar and were no longer fearless warriors.[78] You can draw your own conclusions about this, but it would seem that this may be an early report on the effects of refined sugar on the human body.

HOME INSURANCE POLICY	*The treatment of mental illness should start with a glucose tolerance test to see if the patient can handle sugar*

By the 1700s the sugar and rum industries were so thoroughly tainted by the suffering slaves that the first Anti-Saccharite Society was formed. This humanitarian-minded group lead a boycott of sugar produced by slaves and sought other non-slave produced sources for their own sugar addictions.

In 1812, a Frenchman named Benjamin Delessert invented a way to turn sugar beets into a new kind of sugar loaf, and he was awarded the Legion of Honor by emperor Napoleon.

HOME
INSURANCE
POLICY

> *Why do we eat more sugar and processed foods and less fresh fruits and vegetables? Could we be brainwashed by commercials?*

Can you imagine receiving such a tribute for baking a cake?

Looking at the history of sugar, it's not hard to understand how our values changed as our power of reasoning was replaced by our sweet tooth mentality and economic greed. While the wealth and power of the sugar industries increased, the natural healers, who denounced sugar as a poison, were burned at the stake. And mental illness and sugar related diseases grew in proportion to sugar consumption.

The scourge of sugar continues to this day. Television, radio and newspapers bow to the economic demands of their advertisers—giant food processing companies that use tons and tons of sugar in our food. (Some breakfast cereals are 60% sugar!)

Do you honestly think the media will report on the dangers of sugar when sugar and sugar related industries (i.e., processed foods) are supporting them?

Since it's not fair to condemn sugar without explaining why it's so bad, would you like to know what it does to the human body?

First off, it is nutritionally dead. There is nothing alive in processed, refined sugar. Because it does not provide its own nutrients, Harmony must take vitamins, minerals, and enzymes from other cells in order to prepare sugar for use. In addition, sugar does not produce any ash when it burns.

Now you might think that is good, right?

Wrong. In Chapter 5 we talked about the furnace. When cells work, they naturally create acid. Nutritious food creates alkaline ash when it is burned so acid/alkaline balance is maintained. If the cells are working hard to burn sugar, but the sugar leaves no alkaline ash to neutralize all that acid, what happens to Harmony? The body gets too acidic.

Second, because sugar (sucrose) quickly becomes glucose and is rapidly absorbed, the blood glucose level takes a jump.

HOME
INSURANCE
POLICY

We use sugar laden processed food because it is convenient. The next time you pick up a box of cereal in the grocery store, ask yourself how convenient it is to be sick.

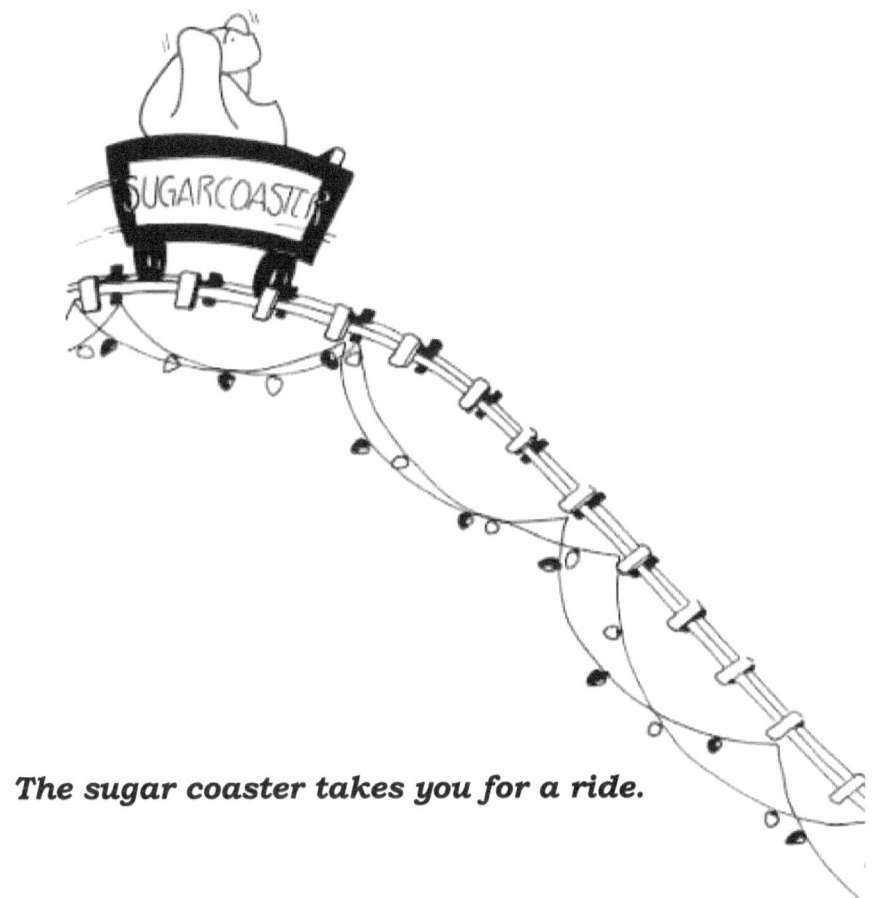

The sugar coaster takes you for a ride.

Although you might think this immediate energy increase feels good, it takes a toll on your body. When the blood glucose level rises this fast, there is not enough oxygen in the blood. When there is not enough oxygen, Harmony is thrown off balance. The pancreas panics and sends insulin to lower the glucose level, while the adrenal glands do just the opposite—they send hormones to keep the level up.

Do you think your hormones enjoy this game of leap-frog?

Newton's Laws teach us that for every action there is an equal and opposite reaction.

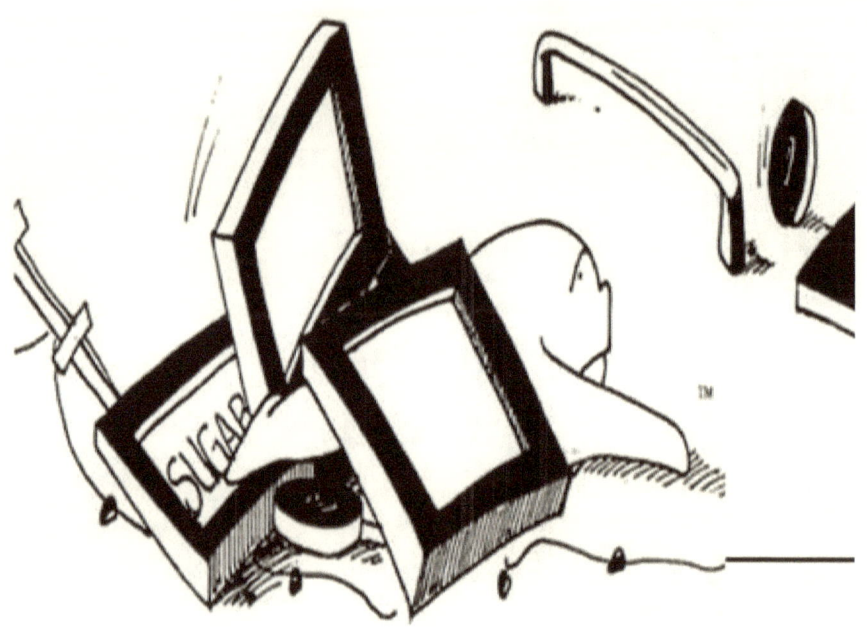

What goes up must come down.

So what happens after that sudden surge in blood glucose? Could it be a sugar coaster crash?

What are some of the sugar related diseases?

Diabetes (more correctly called diabetes mellitus) is probably the most widely recognized. The word *diabetes* is Greek for *passing large volumes of urine. Mellitus* comes from the Latin words *mel* for honey and *itis* for inflammation.

This disease was first described in 1664, by Dr. Thomas Willis, the personal physician to King Charles II. Although Dr. Willis knew the disease was a sugar-induced inflammation, he wisely used the Latin word for honey because the king made huge revenues from the sugar industry.

In those days people could lose their heads if they said anything that offended the royalty.

What would the king have thought if Dr. Willis said, "King, the sugar that is making you rich is killing you."?

HOME INSURANCE POLICY

If you had to choose between health and wealth, which would you choose?

Diabetes can be a deadly disease. Because too much sugar in the blood reduces the amount of oxygen available to the tissues, it is not unusual for a diabetic to lose limbs, which have developed gangrene. Blindness and kidney failure are other effects of this affliction.

Hypoglycemia, low blood sugar, is almost commonplace today. Some health professionals believe that people suffering from hypoglycemia are really allergic to foods, and that elimination of sugar products, both natural and processed, will alleviate their vast array of symptoms.

Another name for hypoglycemia is *idiopathic post-prandial syndrome*. This complicated phrase is more frequently used by medical doctors to describe the symptoms associated with the disorder.

N.I.C.E. (Nutritionally Induced Chronic Endocrinopathy) is a phrase coined by Dr. Jeff Bland, a nutritional biochemist. He claims that hypoglycemia is actually a nutritional or glandular problem that causes blood sugar problems.[79] No matter what name you give this disorder, it is greatly aggravated by the consumption of sugar.

Sugar has also been associated with allergies, arthritis, anxiety, heart disease, and immune problems. It can also cause hyperactivity—especially in children. Candida, a very troubling yeast infection that can be fatal, feeds on sugar.

HOME INSURANCE POLICY

> *Sugar comes from the cane plant—a type of grass. Wheat is also a type of grass. Wheat and long-leaf grasses cause allergies. Do you think that sugar could cause allergies, too?*

If sugar is bad for us, why do we enjoy sweet tasting food so much?

Recent research seems to indicate that even newborn babies prefer sweet tastes, and that our brains may be programmed to select sugary flavors. This could be true because foods that naturally taste sweet tend to provide more energy than bitter foods.[80]

Caffeine is another favorite substance that hurts us while we think it's helping us. If you've ever enjoyed the uplifting surge of a morning cup of coffee, you probably don't want to know what caffeine is really doing to your Harmony.

Home
Insurance
Policy

> *Caffeine is a drug. It is found in coffee, teas, colas, chocolate, and many over-the-counter medicines.*

Research at the School of Medicine at Creighton University in Omaha indicates that long term use of coffee (and more than one cup a day) escalates calcium loss, which intensifies osteoporosis. There is also a tendency among heavy caffeine users to not eat calcium-rich foods. This adds to the problem.

Caffeine is also addictive and can constrict your blood vessels. If you drink coffee every morning before going to work, but suffer headaches when you sleep late on your off days, you just may be addicted to the caffeine. Without that morning fix of blood vessel constrictors, the blood vessels will dilate, causing that aggravating headache or migraine.

Coffee drinking has also been associated with bladder cancer. Caffeine can damage Harmony's genes and this can cause alterations to the DNA. This opens the door to cancer.

Another consequence of high coffee consumption is an increased risk of heart disease. It also raises blood pressure and heart rate, while stimulating the adrenal glands. Because it causes loss of minerals due to its effects on the kidneys, coffee can cause certain degenerative disorders. [81]

HOME INSURANCE POLICY	*Phosphorus in colas and soft drinks robs your bones of calcium.*

Another staple of the American diet is colas, sodas, or soft drinks. These beverages are not only high in sugar and caffeine, they also contain phosphoric acid—to keep those tingling bubbles from going flat. Phosphorus is mixed with sulfuric acid to make this bubble-saving substance.

Because you need twice as much calcium as phosphorus in your blood, when you overload your cells with colas, your body reacts by taking calcium out of your bones in order to reestablish Harmony and balance in your blood.

Smoking is the most deadly substance on Harmony's playground, killing more Americans every year than World Wars I and II and the Viet Nam War combined!

Why would anyone smoke?

When your lungs are full of the thousands of chemicals that make up tobacco smoke there is not enough room for oxygen. Harmony cannot live without oxygen!

Side stream smoke is also a killer. Smoke exhaled from a smoker's lungs is even more polluted with all the garbage the smoker has accumulated, and the smoke that comes from the end of the cigarette that is lit is more toxic than the smoke inhaled.

Some of the diseases and health problems caused by smoking are:

- Lung cancer,
- Emphysema,
- Chronic bronchitis,
- Altered immune system,
- Low birth-weight babies of smoking mothers,
- Heart disease, and
- Peptic ulcer disease.

Our government spends millions of dollars on tobacco subsidies each year.

Why? Tobacco is a killer, plain and simple.

We imprison distributors of heroin and marijuana. We imprison intoxicated drivers. Smoking is the Number One Killer in this country. Why don't we put the killers in jail?

President Jimmy Carter summed it up in 1986 when he said, "I think there is a deliberate commitment on the part of the tobacco industry to cause death for profit." [82]

When you take Harmony to the playground, and the only playmates are sugar, caffeine, and nicotine, you're playing a deadly game.

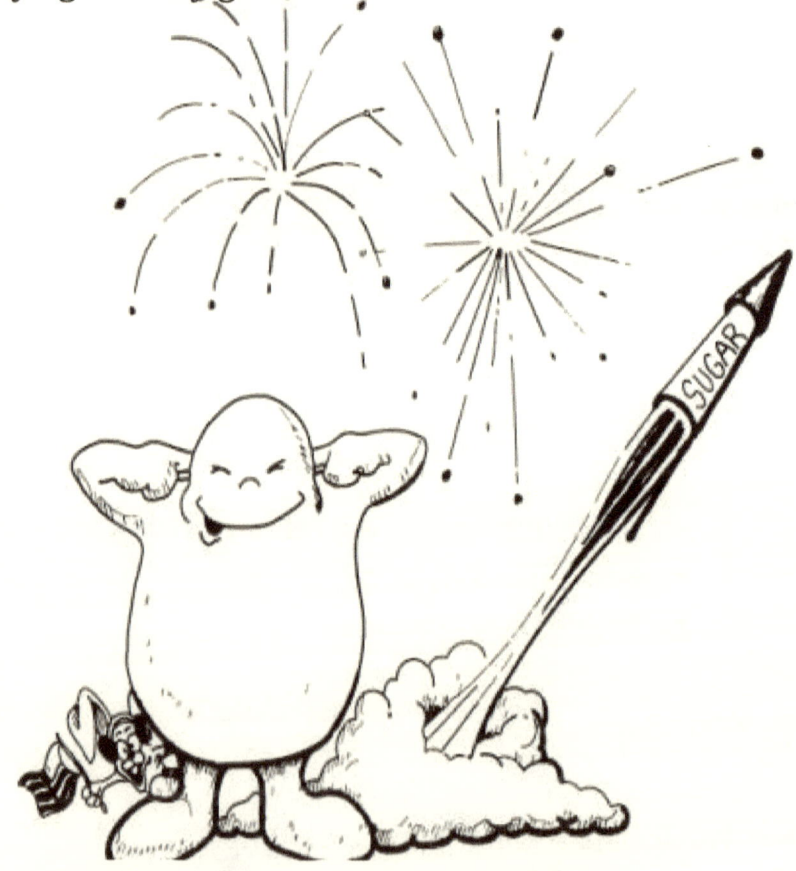

Declare your independence from sugar.

Chapter 12

The Siding

The siding on the house protects the occupants from scorching summer sun, freezing winter snow, and raging thunderstorms. It also gives the house direct and immediate contact with the surrounding environment. When you build a house you need more siding than any other component.

Your skin is the *siding* of your home. It is the largest organ of your body! Skin is your body's first contact with everything you encounter, and it doesn't hesitate to convey what is going on around you. It tells you the sun is hot, snow is cold, rain is wet. Your skin also communicates emotional messages. The delicate kiss of a child, warm embrace of an old friend, or tender touch of a lover all create physical and emotional reactions inside our bodies that start with an event experienced by our skin.

The siding of your house is also your first defense against germs and other harmful substances in the environment. If your skin is intact, the only way germs can enter your body is through openings, such as the nose, mouth or

eyes. Dr. Earl Mindell says, "the mildly acidic film of oil
and sweat which coats the skin is itself slightly harmful
to bacteria and fungus."[83] So you can see that your skin
is a very important part of your immune system because
it's your body's first line of defense.

Skin is also a major member of your house cleaning team
because it regularly and readily eliminates toxins that
accumulate inside your body. Millions of sweat glands in
your skin excrete waste products, excess mineral salts[84]
and water, and many health professionals call skin *the
second kidney.* The days you don't exercise, you'll
eliminate about a pint of these toxins. But when you
engage in a strenuous workout, you can get up to eight
quarts of these trouble-makers out of your house in one
day!

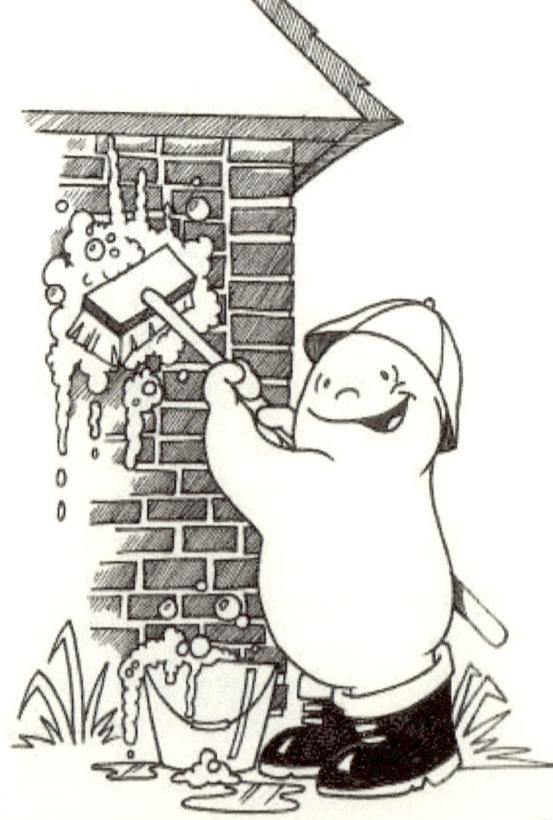

Because we can't look inside our bodies daily to evaluate our degree of health or illness, our skin can be a very valuable guide to wellness.

What do you see when you look in the mirror?

HOME
INSURANCE | *Your mirror can tell you a lot about your health.*
POLICY

Here's a short list of some typical skin problems and what they can indicate:

♦ Acne, pimples and blemishes—gland and hormone imbalances, too much fat in the diet, deficiency of essential fatty acids, over-indulgence in sugar consumption, not enough green vegetables in the diet, stress;

♦ Boils and carbuncles—systemic toxicity, viral infection, staph infection due to high acid condition;

♦ Canker and cold sores—B-complex deficiency, herpes simplex virus, sensitivity to gluten, high-acid diet, chronic viral infection;

♦ Callouses and corns—kidney malfunction; too much caffeine, sugar, or saturated fat; poor elimination of calcium;

◆ Dark circles under the eyes—iron deficiency, chronic allergies, or liver or kidney malfunction;

◆ Dandruff and Seborrhea—consuming too much alcohol, saturated fats, sugars or starches; shortage of essential fatty acids, green vegetables; sensitivity to hair dyes;

◆ Dermatitis—deficiency in essential fatty acids, eating too many acid forming foods, poor liver function, stress;

◆ Eczema—diabetes, asthma, or candida albicans; hypersensitivity to cow's milk, eggs, tomatoes, artificial colors and food preservatives;

◆ Plantar warts—insufficient stomach acid (HCL), constipation or toxemia due to high fat and refined carbohydrate diet; not enough vegetable source protein;

◆ Psoriasis—arthritis or an underactive thyroid gland;

◆ Shingles—allergy to milk, shellfish, wheat, MSG, artificial food additives such as preservatives; drinking chlorinated water; liver or adrenal gland problems, prescription drugs;

◆ Warts and moles—insufficient Vitamin A and minerals, viral infection, over-use of antibiotics, immunity depressed by vaccination.

As you can see, skin reflects our state of health. When we have any of the above skin conditions, our bodies are waving red flags at us. If we ignore these minor repair orders we may have to get a major overhaul in the future.

HOME
INSURANCE
POLICY[85]

> *Skin problems are one of the surest signs of poor nutrition.*   - Dr. Linda G. Rector-Page

There are three major determinants for healthy skin. Let's list them in order or importance:

1. Nutrients you bring in the front door;

2. Limited exposure to sun; and

3. Natural skin care products.

Why would we put nutrients first?

Because you are what you eat and healthy skin is created inside your body, then migrates to the outside. In a normal life span, you will manufacture about 40 pounds of skin for the siding of your home. Your current supply probably weighs about six pounds.

Your skin has two basic parts, the epidermis and the dermis.

The epidermis is the outside of your home—it's the part you wash in your morning shower or evening bath.
It has three primary layers, and combined, they create about 20 layers of cells:

♦ The paper thin surface layer would measure about 20 square feet if you could stretch it out. It is composed of keratin, scaly dead cells.

♦ New skin cells make up the middle layer. These cells are constantly moving to the surface to replace the dead cells which are continuously sloughed off.

♦ Through cell division, the basal layer provides new cells which migrate to the surface. Melanin (pigment) in the basal layer gives your skin its color.

You might think of the dermis as your house-wrap—that extra layer of protection for your home between the exterior siding the interior insulation

The dermis encloses working parts for the skin system: Hair follicles, sweat glands, blood vessels, lymph channels, muscle cells, sebaceous (oil-producing) glands, and nerve fibers which give you the sense of touch so you'll know if an object is hot or cold, hard or soft, smooth or prickly, etc.

The dermis, about four times as thick as the epidermis, makes your skin strong and flexible. Deterioration of the dermis causes wrinkling. A layer of new skin cells cover the dermis.

Underneath the dermis is a layer of fat called the subcutis or subcutaneous fat. This is the insulation for Harmony's home. When the dermis breaks down due to injury, aging, or poor nutrition, this fatty tissue moves into a more visible position under the skin. We call this unattractive, dimpled condition cellulitis.

Sebaceous glands empty a special oil they produce into hair follicles (we'll talk more about hair in Chapter 13). This sebum is a waterproof oil that lubricates your skin to help it retain water. Remember, your body is about 75% water. When you lose too much H_2O, your skin becomes dry and flaky.

HOME
INSURANCE
POLICY

Well-hydrated skin is supple and healthy

Most of the sebaceous glands are on your face. Other concentrations of these glands are found on the back, chest, and shoulders. When these glands get over-productive (usually due to hormonal changes during puberty or poor diet) the openings can get clogged. This causes acne.

Two types of sweat glands deliver their cargo to the two million pores in your skin. The eccrine sweat glands work hard when you exercise to eliminate water and mineral salts. This moisture, called perspiration, then evaporates and you cool down. Because one of these salts is sodium chloride, your sweat tastes salty. High temperatures and stress also make the eccrine glands work more.

Have you ever noticed an odor under your arms or in the genital area?

If you don't like it, blame your apocrine sweat glands, which are located in these areas. These glands not only release water and salts, they also eliminate wastes that contain nitrogen. Odor is created when this discharge is mixed with bacteria on the skin's surface.

HOME
INSURANCE
POLICY[86]

> *Toxins are expelled through the skin, which needs to be kept clean and scrubbed ...*
> - Louise Tenney, M.H.

If you were building a brick house you would use mortar to hold the bricks in place. Wood siding would be held in place with nails. The mortar and nails for Harmony's house are two proteins called collagen and elastin.

Harmony's house has more collagen than any other protein because it's also a component of connective tissue. Connective tissue fastens one type of body part to another, such as a tendon to bone or a ligament to muscle. Collagen forms fibers which provide strength, flexibility and support of the skin.

Elastin, as the name implies, gives your skin its supple, elastic features. This protein fiber, together with collagen, creates skin tone and resilience.

HOME
INSURANCE
POLICY[87]

> *A nutrient deficient diet is a major source of skin afflictions*

You can easily see that Harmony must maintain collagen and elastin if you are to have beautiful, healthy skin. But you can't do this job by putting creams and lotions on the outside of the house.

For one thing, your skin can't absorb collagen. It can only get this essential ingredient from its own internal manufacturing plant. Because the other components of healthy skin are also built on the inside of the house, here is a list of nutrients Harmony needs for the siding of your home:

♦ Vitamin C; you can't make collagen without it.

♦ Copper, to synthesize collagen and elastin.

♦ Omega 3 fatty acids, essential for proper cell function, including your skin cells.

♦ Silica/Silicon, a major component of collagen, found in our blood in the same concentration as in sea water. "Some researchers speculate that a decline in silicon levels in the body contributes significantly to the aging process."[88]

- ◆ Zinc, to repair and build new skin tissue.

- ◆ Glucosamine, formulated from glucose and amino acids by your body; it's an essential building block for tissue between skin cells and mucous membranes.

- ◆ Water, to keep skin properly moisturized and flush toxins—a source of blemishes—out of the body.

- ◆ Biotin, to prevent dry skin, which enhances the appearance of wrinkles.

- ◆ Riboflavin, to prevent dry, cracked lips.

- ◆ Selenium, to prevent free radical damage, a major cause of skin aging.

- ◆ Beta-carotene, a non-toxic precursor for Vitamin A, helps relieve skin problems.

- ◆ Vitamin E, one of the antioxidants, an anti-aging nutrient.

HOME
INSURANCE
POLICY[89]

| *If you've been neglecting your health, under extra stress and unable to sleep well, your skin will let the world know.*- Susan Smith Jones, Ph.D. |

Now that we've talked about the functions of the largest organ, and nutrients needed inside the house to maintain the skin, let's step outside and take a look at the sun.

We could not exist without the sun. You might say it's the essential nutrient for Mother Earth. It also provides us with Vitamin D, which is one of our essential nutrients. This splendid process takes place when the sun's ultraviolet rays make contact with your body and convert a form of cholesterol found in the skin into Vitamin D. For this reason we frequently call Vitamin D the *sunshine vitamin.*

Fresh air and sunshine also have positive effects on our psyche. There's nothing like a brisk walk on a bright day to bring you out of the doldrums. There are even some people who become depressed during the short days of winter because they don't get enough exposure to the sun.

So we all need sunshine. It's good for us both physically and mentally. But somehow, a number of years ago, many light skinned people got the strange notion that tanned skin was a sign of good health. Nothing could be further from the truth!

As these ill advised people took to beaches, pool decks, and tanning salons in search of the perfect tan, the rate of skin cancer rose along with premature aging of the skin. Science has now proven that overexposure to sun breaks down collagen and elastin. When you destroy the mortar and nails that hold the siding on Harmony's house, the skin loses its support system. Without support, it sags and wrinkles. Even the American Academy of Dermatology has said that wrinkles are mostly caused by sun and not age.

You may want to protest these statements by saying you use sunscreen and you're protected. So let's take a look at the real culprit in this discussion.

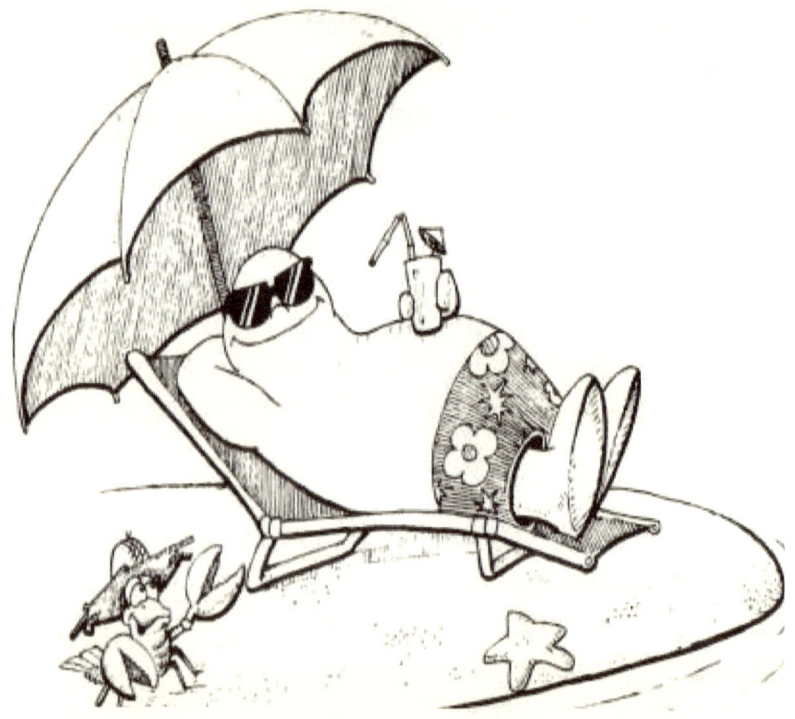

Don't overexpose Harmony

The sun emits two types of ultraviolet (UV) light: UVA and UVB. The UVA rays are the longest and most abundant but they have a lower intensity. Therefore, you don't feel them. There are fewer UVB rays, and they are shorter, but they are much more intense. It is these short, intense UVB rays that burn the skin. When you put sunscreen on your skin, you are protecting it from the UVB rays only.

Guess what?

The UVA rays, which do not burn because of their low intensity, penetrate to the very deepest layers of your skin. That means it gets to those precious proteins, collagen and elastin. This happens year round, regardless of season. It even gets through on cloudy, foggy, or smoggy days.

How do you think you would feel if you were just a little protein molecule that was constantly bombarded by UV rays?

HOME INSURANCE POLICY	*Sun exposure can be dangerously magnified by some medications. If you're on a pharmaceutical drug and want to get in the sun, be sure to check with your pharmacist first.*

Let's take a break from the sun and go shopping at the largest department store at the local mall.

What's the first thing you generally encounter?

The cosmetic department, right?

Everywhere you look, beautiful women are enticing you to try their products. The next time you want to talk yourself out of an expensive purchase, just take a look at the label. If it contains any of the following synthetic ingredients used for preservatives, microbial growth inhibitors, humectants, foaming agents, softeners, colors, fragrances, or pH adjusters you don't want it:

☒ Imidazolidinyl and diazolindiyl ureas; methyl, propyl, butyl or ethyl parabens; petrolatum; propylene glycol; PVP/VA copolymer; sodium lauryl sulfate; stearalkonium chloride; or triethanolamine.

Just because you don't ingest these potentially harmful synthetic products does not mean they are safe.

Remember those two million pores we talked about?

Well, they can funnel things into the body just as easily as they empty out toxins, water and salts. Research indicates that many of these artificial substances are carcinogenic.

Propylene glycol and sodium lauryl sulfate have been associated with kidney damage and eye problems in children who were exposed to them through shampoos.

You should also be wary of *all natural* cosmetics and skin care products. Many of these do indeed have natural base ingredients but use synthetics for preservation and shelf life.

Mother Nature has provided many plants, spices, vegetables and herbs for care of the skin. Here are a few of them:

Aloe vera, widely recognized for its effectiveness in treating burns; a soothing antibiotic; stimulates cell growth.

Clove extract, an excellent germicide; oil from young plants is a good stimulant.

Dandelion, good for acne and eczema.

Elder flower, the herbalists cosmetic since every part of the plant is said to aid the complexion; soothes skin and bleaches freckles.

Eyebright, cooling and detoxifying; an excellent remedy for eye problems such as inflammation, conjunctivitis and ulcers.

Jojoba oil, because it mimics sebum, it is an effective moisturizer.

Lemon grass, a natural astringent; used on insect bites and as warm poultice on boils.

Marigold tincture, effective treatment for bruises, sprains, ulcers, and bad scars.

Marshmallow root, heals inflammation and prevents infections such as gangrene.

Myrrh, when mixed with **goldenseal**, makes a healing antiseptic salve.

Nettle leaves, a good treatment for eczema and other skin ailments.

Papaya seed paste, for skin diseases such as ringworm; the juice dissolves corns, warts, and pimples.

Red clover, used by Indians for sore eyes and in salve for burns.

Redmond Clay, for stings, bug bites, and beauty marks.

Rosemary, a skin stimulant; used to treat open sores, bites and stings.

Sage, in lotion form, heals sores, skin eruptions; stops wound bleeding.

Thyme, a powerful antiseptic, destroys fungal infections such as athlete's feet and skin parasites, crabs and lice.

Watercress leaves juice, put on face to treat freckles and pimples.

White oak bark, is a strong astringent, and an excellent cleanser.

Witch hazel, good for burns, insect bites, and bleeding wounds.

Yellow dock, an astringent and blood purifier, treats chronic skin problems.

Yucca, for skin disorders, was used by Southwest Indians to stop bleeding and prevent inflammation.

As you can see, everything we could possibly need or want for healthy skin has been provided by Mother Nature.

In his book, *The Joy of Life*, Dr. Elliot M. Goldway splendidly describes skin:

> *Imagine a material that is waterproof, like tarpaulin, yet can let out water and oil; that can protect like a suit of armor, and yet is infinitely sensitive to touch; that remains firm, yet is more flexible than rubber. It is also a beautiful material—whether pink and white, brown, black or yellow.*[90]

Your skin covers you like the siding on a house and it faithfully provides you with information you need to survive each moment of your life. If you want to live in the state of wellness, you'll provide your skin with proper nutrients, shield it from too much sun, and be mindful of what you put on it—because you can't live without it.

Chapter 13

The Roof

Have you ever noticed the vast variety of roofing materials and how they affect the appearance of a house?

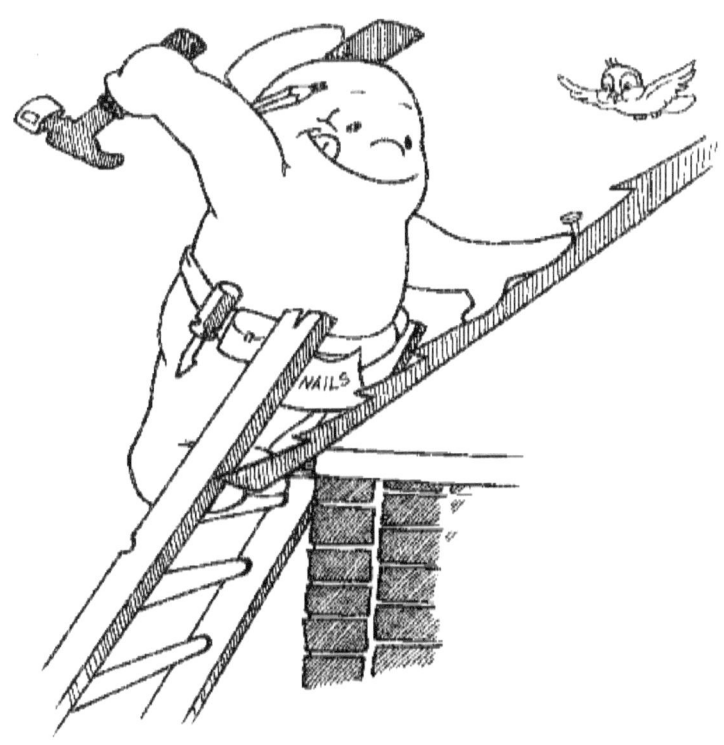

Roofing comes in all sorts of shapes, sizes and colors. Some are wood, others are asphalt. In third world countries you'll see mud roofs, and thatched roofs in England are treasured. The newest trend in roofing is standing seam sheet metal or steel. No matter what the texture or color, the roof seems to make a statement about the overall condition of the house.

The hair on your head is the roof of Harmony's house and it says a lot about the condition of your home. Like skin, your hair is a direct reflection of your health, telling us if you are well-nourished or nutrient deficient. Hair analysis can determine the amount of minerals or toxic metals you have in your home.

Right or wrong, we also tend to describe a person's personality by their hair color. How often have you said someone was *a dumb blond* or *hot tempered redhead.* If your hair is dull or plain, you could be *mousey.* When describing yourself, your hair is probably one of the first things you'll mention.

Hair speaks loudly about who we are and there are several Biblical references to it. Do you remember the story of Sampson? His strength was attributed to his hair!

Here are a few other Biblical references to hair:

> *And the very hairs of your head are all numbered.*
> -Matthew 10:30

*For women are proud of their long hair, while a man
with long hair tends to be ashamed.*
                                    - I Corinthians, 11:15.

*He cut his hair only once a year—and then only
because it weighed three pounds and was too much
of a load to carry around.* - II Samuel, 14:26.

The average person has about 100,000 hairs on their
head and loses 50 to 100 of these daily. Each hair grows
out of a follicle surrounded by a bulb. These bulbs each
receive nutrients from the blood which must be supplied
to every single one of them. That's why good circulation is
essential for proper hair development.

HOME INSURANCE POLICY	*The condition of the shingles on your roof is directly related to the nutrients you invite into your home.*

The color of your hair is determined by the melanin
inside the follicle. When your melanin production slows
down, your hair will turn grey. If you completely stop
producing this pigment, your hair will be white.

There are three parts to the hair shaft: the medulla,
cortex and cuticle. The medulla is the center core. It is
surrounded by the cortex, which is somewhat thicker.
Surrounding the outside is the tough cuticle.

The shape of your hair shaft determines whether your hair will be straight, wavy, or curly. A round shaft produces straight hair; curved shafts create wavy hair; and a kidney shaped shaft makes curly hair. These hairs will last anywhere from two to six years and grow about half an inch a month. That's good news if you just got a bad haircut.

Although we emphasize hair's appearance, the roof on the house really has several important functions. Hair not only shields your scalp from exposure to sun and wind, it also provides a nice cushion for your scull. The hairs that line your eyelids (lashes), and fine hairs in your nose, strain the air and filter out particles such as dirt and dust. These are good reasons to take care of your hair.

Dr. Linda Rector-Page has a description of hair that fits right in with our roof model for the covering of your home:

> In healthy hair, the cell walls of the hair cuticle
> lie flat like shingles, leaving hair soft and shiny.
> In damaged or dry hair, the cuticle shingles are
> broken and create gaps that make hair porous
> and dull.[91]

If you have dull, lifeless hair, hair loss, brittle or breaking hair, you have probably:

♦   Failed to provide the proper nutrients to grow good hair, which means your body is deficient in other areas as well;

♦   Experienced an illness or internal exposure to toxic substances such as chemotherapy or radiation; or

♦   Damaged your hair with overexposure to sun, environmental pollutants, or hair treatment products such as dyes, perms, or straighteners.

Let's take a look at proper hair nutrition so you can build a good roof for your home.

Your hair is 98% protein; this is your number one nutrient. But don't start loading up on acid-forming high protein meats. For one thing, too much acid will deplete calcium, a component of healthy hair. For another, "hair loss is associated with a high fat diet."[92] Since animal products are the only source of fat, get your proteins from vegetables, beans and soy.

If your diet does not have enough of these nutrients, you can't produce a head full of healthy hair:

Vitamins - A, B, C and E;

Minerals - zinc, iron, selenium and silica/silicon; and

Cysteine, an Amino acid.

Deficiencies in B12 and pantothenic acid (B5) can cause graying; insufficient EFA's (essential fatty acids) can make your hair dry.

Remember, consult your health professional if you want to increase your intake of these nutrients. Diabetics or people allergic to MSG (monosodium glutamate) should not take cysteine, and too much iron can cause other problems, including destructive oxidation.

If you don't have enough shingles on your roof you should look at your diet. Two commonly consumed hair robbers are salt and sugar. Cut back on these if you are experiencing hair loss.

HOME
INSURANCE
POLICY

> *Salt and sugar are home wreckers—and they'll even steal the shingles right off your roof.*

Pharmaceutical drugs can also be antagonist to normal hair growth, especially birth control pills, antibiotics, anticoagulants, and prescriptions for high blood pressure. Needless to say, chemo-therapy, a systemic poison that gets into every room in your house, causes massive loss of essential nutrients which leads to hair loss.

Since hair mirrors our inner health, here is a list of some ailments that can cause hair problems:

Anemia

Celiac disease (wheat gluten intolerance)

Diabetes

Eczema and psoriasis

Emotional stress and/or anxiety

Liver malfunction

Low calorie diets (deplete biotin)

Lupus and other auto-immune diseases

Menopause (too much estrogen or too little progesterone)

Ovarian or adrenal tumors

Surgery

Thyroid gland imbalance

Now that we know what nutrients we need to build a good roof, and the diseases that can damage our shingles, let's look at some outside causes for hair problems:

Sun

Pollutants, and

Hair treatment products.

Excessive sun can dehydrate the hair, stripping it of natural moisture, leaving it dry and brittle. Another danger of too much sun is scalp damage. If your hair is not thick, you could even sunburn your scalp.

Like the skin, your hair can also funnel harmful ingredients into your house, right through that roof and into the attic. There are potentially thousands of synthetic chemical combinations used to preserve hair products, inhibit bacteria, add aroma, adjust pH, enhance color, increase foaming action, condition, and moisturize. Here's a few you will want to avoid:

- Stearalkonium chloride - originally developed as a fabric softener, this chemical supposedly conditions hair. Unfortunately, it is toxic and can cause allergic reactions.

- Formaldehyde – a known carcinogen, frequently used in hair products. According to Stacy Malkan, co-founder of the Campaign for Safe Cosmetics and author of *Not Just a Pretty Face: The Ugly Side of the Beauty Industry* "Formaldehyde is a known human carcinogen and it shouldn't be allowed in hair products, period,"[93]

- Cocoamide DEA – a hair detergent, inhibits fetal brain development.[94]

- Artificial colors – generally manufactured from coal tar, which has heavy metal salts. You never want heavy metals in your body or on your skin or hair. Heavy metals include arsenic, cadmium, lead, and mercury.

- Parabens – disrupt endocrine function, and play a role in breast cancer and decreased fertility in men.

- Ethoxylates – a type of emulsifier, damages DNA.

With more than 500 chemicals just in hair and nail products, we can't begin to list all the side effects. But if you are aware that they are not safe, you can be diligent about your personal home and use only the natural products that will keep your roof in good shape.

CHAPTER 14

The Backyard Shade Tree

A visit to your home would not be complete without a stop in the backyard. As a child you probably found the backyard a wonderful place to explore nature, play games, or just wile away a lazy afternoon swinging in the old hammock. Regardless of the activity, times like these were always good for getting in touch with your higher self and reclaiming a sense of peace.

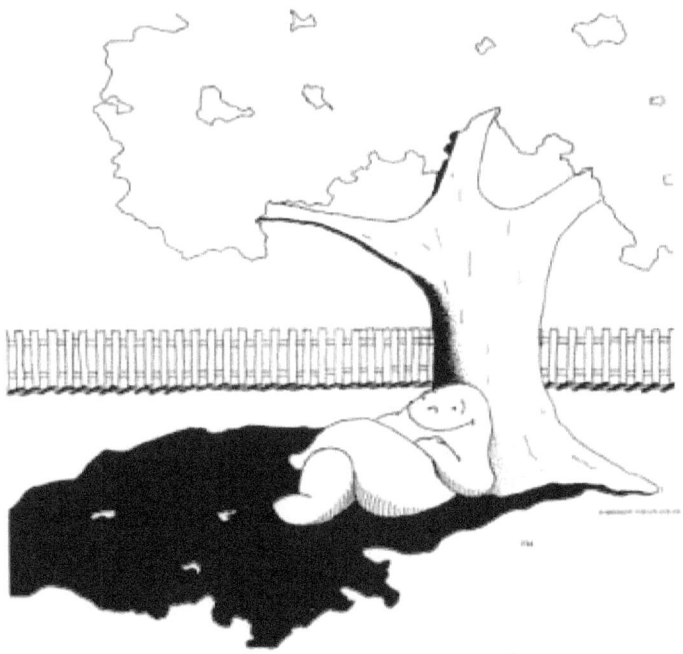

As adults we are frequently so engrossed with other activities in life that we seldom set aside time to just enjoy the fact that we are alive. Over burdened with incomes to earn, bills to pay, errands to run, and chores to do, we end up in the State of Stress and wonder how we missed the Train to Wellness.

Your mind is the most wondrous creation in all of nature, but it still needs proper nutritional habits if it is to work at an optimum level of performance. Because the mind is the center of our being, and can directly affect every aspect of our lives—physical, mental, emotional and spiritual—it is crucial to our well being that we take proper care of it. The very nature of the mind leads us to believe that because it is not a purely physical part of us it does not require any special attention.

But the mind is the home of the real you! It houses your thoughts, your feelings, and your emotions. It not only controls your bodily functions, it is the very center of everything you experience in life. Perceptions formed in your mind determine how you respond to every stimulus you encounter, whether good or bad.

HOME
INSURANCE
POLICY

If negative thoughts create negative responses in our bodies, what do positive thoughts create?

You've heard the expression, "just kick back and relax." Have you ever followed this worthy advice? If not, why? Do you know how to relax?

Why is relaxation important, anyway?

If you are truly on the road to wellness you will find that eliminating stress is not a far-fetched idea but rather an integral part of your new lifestyle and a new you. Even if you have taken the steps to improve your health and your life by modifying your eating habits to include wholesome, nutritious, natural foods, even if you have started a regular exercise program, and even if you have discovered alternative therapies for illness that help you to heal yourself, your journey to the State of Wellness will not be completed if you still have too much stress in your life. Relaxation and meditation are nutrition for your mind!

HOME INSURANCE POLICY	*It is neither wealth nor splendor, but tranquility and occupation, which give happiness.* - Thomas Jefferson

There are many forms of stress. Much of it is unavoidable but a certain amount can be desirable. Stress can be the driving force that propels us to meet the demands of job and family. The result of this type of stress can be the inner satisfaction of a life well lived. Stress can also be a major life crisis, such as a death or divorce, that generates anxiety or emotional pain.

We all live with stress every day—getting yelled at by the boss, sitting in traffic on the freeway, or trying to eat dinner in a restaurant next to a couple with a screaming child or talking loudly on a cell phone. Day to day routines that we repeat over and over, week in and week out, without pause or reflection, can mean we have gotten ourselves in a rut. Being in an endless rut can create an endless stream of stress on the body.

HOME INSURANCE POLICY	*Avoid getting in ruts. Ruts are graves with the ends knocked out.*

Making decisions, balancing the checkbook, job interviews—the list of stressors in modern American life is endless. In the long run, it's not the type of stress we undergo that undermines our health. Our response to stress ruins our health. The response starts in our minds.

While many of us thrive on certain stressors, if we continually react with the *fight or flight response*, over a period of time we will lose our way to the state of wellness. Stress can aggravate any existing health problem and create others, just to name a few:

✓ Headaches,

✓ Stomach ulcers,

✓ High blood pressure,

✓ Insomnia,

✓ Emotional imbalance,

✓ Eating disorders, and

✓ Lowed immunity.

Although you may not be able to control the stressors in your life, you can control your response by controlling your mind. If you control your mind, you will have the ability to greatly alleviate many of the negative effects of the typical American lifestyle. When stress is eliminated, you can restore Harmony to your home.

HOME INSURANCE POLICY	*He that would live in peace and at ease, must not speak all he knows, nor judge all he sees.* - Anonymous

What are some methods for controlling your response to stress or eliminating its affects?

Many techniques employ the mind—that indescribable realm of human existence that can change not only our emotions and psychological health, but our physical bodies as well.

My mother taught me the powerful effect of her mind on her body. She was a gifted artist who specialized in scientific illustrations that were generally recognized as the best in her field. In her sixties she fell and broke her right arm in nine places, completely disabling her drawing hand.

When I was called to the emergency room at the hospital, our family doctor said, "She'll never draw again. The nerve damage is too extensive. We'll be lucky if she can regain enough function for even limited use of it."

I said, "Well don't tell Mother that she'll never draw again. Art is her life. It would kill her."

No one was allowed to mention to my mom that she would never draw again, but everyone who visited her was told to tell the distraught artist that she would be drawing again soon.

After the cast was removed, she started a grueling physical rehabilitation program, constantly encouraged by her children and co-workers. Ten weeks after the accident that should have ended her career, she was back at the drawing board, producing some of the finest work that she had ever done. Mother was the artist who drew my New Life butterfly—many years after her accident.

Years later I lost almost all use of both arms due to a bulging disc in my neck caused by an extremely stressful situation in my life. At the time I was a construction secretary, but could not feel the typewriter keys under my fingers. Normal tasks, like opening doors or pushing the vacuum cleaner, were impossible. During my two-year road to complete recovery—without surgery—I kept remembering my mother's ordeal.

"I can get better. I will get better," I told myself over and over every day. Today I am a writer and spend up to 18 hours a day at my computer.

HOME
INSURANCE
POLICY

> *Your mind is the most powerful possession you will ever have. You can do anything if you think you can.*

There are many ways you can use your incredible mind to eliminate stress and these are just a few of them:

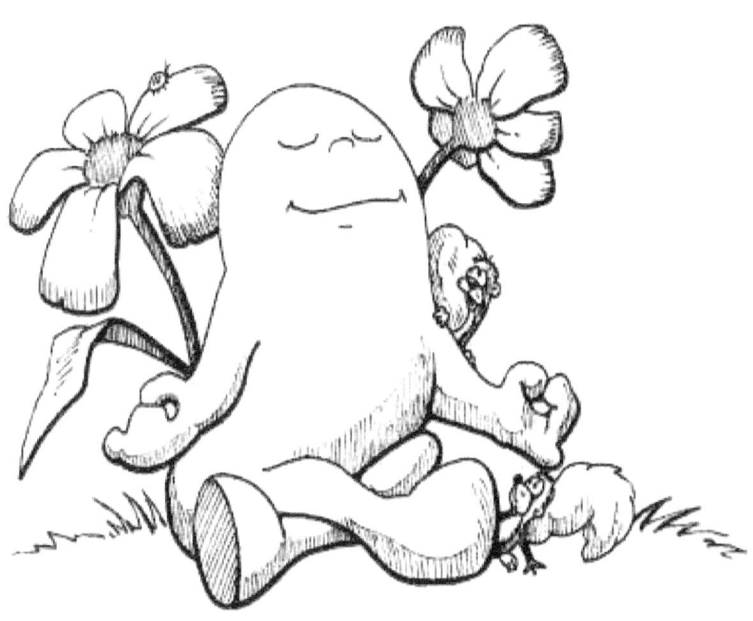

Meditation is a mental exercise that trains your mind to tap into a higher level of awareness. By getting in touch with your higher self you can use your mind in marvelous ways.

You can use mediation to disconnect from the world and find a few moments of peace. Many of us think that people who meditate are doing so in order to withdraw from the world. In truth, after meditating, you will find that you are even more connected to the world in which you live. The difference is that it creates peace, and you can call up this peace whenever you need it.

Visualization uses mental imagery to create positive situations in your life. It is not unusual for star athletes to use creative visualizations as part of their training routine. They actively work at *seeing* themselves performing at their peak ability and then do precisely that on the day of competition. By eliminating apprehensions about your performance, you can reduce the amount of stress in your life.

Self-hypnosis can be used for pain control and reinforcement of other therapeutic treatments done by a licensed hypnotherapist. Women in childbirth have found it an effective and painless way to deliver. Many who suffer from chronic pain such as arthritis use self-hypnosis rather than drugs to treat ailments. Relief from pain is another stress reducer.

Autogenics (AT) combines techniques used in meditation and self-hypnosis to reduce stress. Following a designated training ritual, people using AT get into a light trance, followed by specific instructions for improvement of problems such as excessive weight, depression, headaches, allergies, and anxiety.

Dream analysis can help us unlock inner feelings and get in touch with hidden areas in our lives that may be creating unconscious stress. Dreams can help us discover answers to problems and give us new insights that encourage us to take specific actions or methods to resolve conflicts. Because dreams are the unique creation of the dreamer, if the interpretation you put to a dream feels good, or seems to click, you've probably got the right answer. Learning to recognize conflicts and their solutions presented in dreams can be a powerful weapon of the mind to eliminate stress.

HOME INSURANCE POLICY	*Your body is the baggage you must carry through life. The more excess baggage, the shorter the trip.* - Arnold H. Glasow

Relaxation, like proper nutrition, is not an option. It is just one of the steps each of us must take if we are to reach the State of Wellness. The path to wellness may not always be easy, but given time and effort, you will be richly rewarded. The essential keys to Harmony in your home will always include:

- Proper Nutrition
- Stimulating Exercise
- Natural Therapies
- Nutritional Supplements
- Stress Reduction

If you want to live in a state of wellness where disease is outlawed, arm yourself with good nutritional habits. Remember that wellness is more than just the absence of illness. Even if you are not well now, it is never too late to take the first step on the path that will lead to a new life. When you have achieved wellness, your physical body will function normally; you will be mentally alert and spiritually attuned to the world, and your place in it. Every activity can become a source of pleasure, and you can enjoy life in new ways.

As we said in the beginning of this book, your body is the most precious home you will ever have.

Be mindful of the guests you invite into your home; keep your pantry well stocked with the essential nutrients, and stoke your furnace with the proper combination of proteins, carbohydrates, and fat.

Make regular use of the workout room, and be sure to check out the contents of your own medicine cabinet if you don't feel well.

Keep your home secured with ample supplies of anti-oxidants, and stay away from the toxic playground as much as possible.

Last, and possibly the most important reminder of all, take daily trips to your backyard shade tree; lie back in the hammock and use your incredible mind to envision pictures in the clouds, floating in the vast blue sky.

Thank the Beneficent Creator for giving you seventy five trillion chances to have Harmony in your life.

Embrace yourself, love yourself, and take care of your home. For you are truly a beautiful, unique and amazing creation!

HOME
INSURANCE
POLICY

Nothing changes until you do.

                                    - Jack Clarke

You will find, as you look back upon your life, that the moments that stand out, the moments when you have really lived, are the moments when you have done things in the spirit of love.

- Henry Drummond

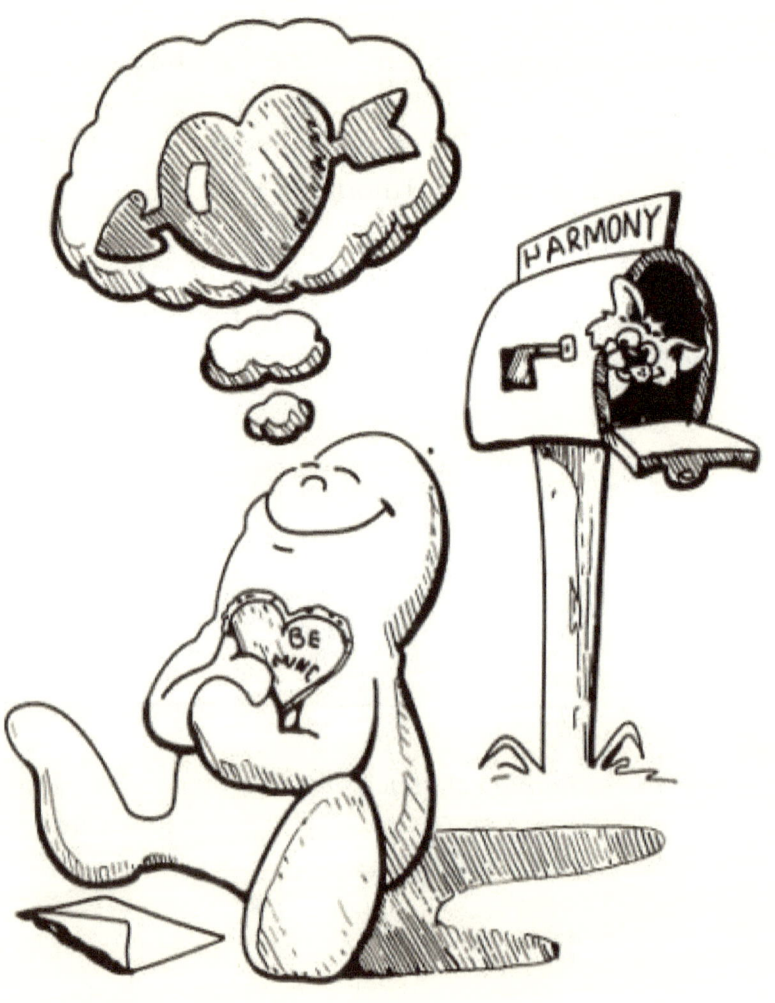

We are much more
than what we eat,
but what we eat
can make us much more
than what we are.

\- Adele Davis

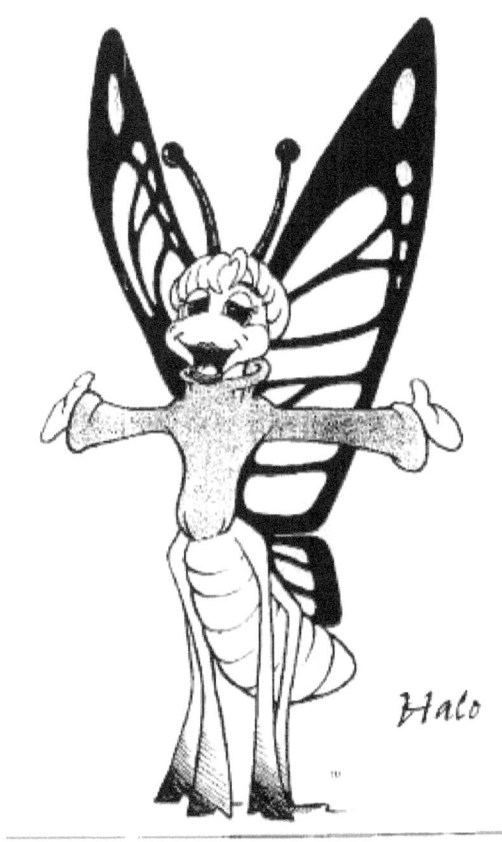

HERBS

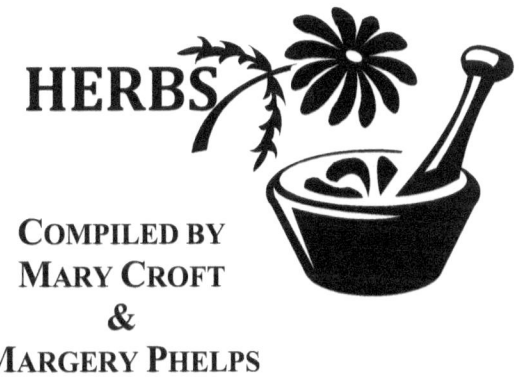

COMPILED BY
MARY CROFT
&
MARGERY PHELPS

For the earth which drinks in the rain that often comes upon it, and bears herbs useful for those by whom it is cultivated receives blessings from God. - Hebrews 6:7

Alfalfa - A good source of Vitamin A, it is very helpful in reducing fevers. It acts as a blood purifier and contains natural fluoride.

Astragalus - From China, this herb supports T-cell function and is a great strengthener of the immune system. It aids adrenal function, lowers blood pressure, and improves circulation, thus promoting healing of damaged tissues.

Black Cohosh - From the same family as the buttercup and peony, it is an excellent sedative for the central nervous system. Since it contains a natural estrogen, it is helpful with menopausal hot flashes. *Black* originates from its dark roots, and *cohosh* is Algonquian for *rough*.

Native Americans used it for fatigue, sore throat, arthritis and rattlesnake bite, hence it is also referred to as snake root.

Bladderwrack - Used for treating goiter, for many years this variety of seaweed was the only source for iodine. A metabolic stimulant, it is often part of a weight reducing program. It is also helpful in relieving arthritic and rheumatic problems.

Brigham Tea - see Ephedra.

Buckthorn Bark - Non-habit forming and non-irritable, it keeps the bowels regular.

Burdock - Very high in nutrition, the root of this plant is used by the Japanese as a vegetable. Considered a hormone-balancing herb, it removes toxins from the body and aids digestion and hemorrhoids. It contains chemicals that kill bacteria and fungi that cause disease.

Chamomile - This flower makes a good tea and is excellent for a nervous stomach. It has been found to relieve cramping associated with the menstrual cycle.

Cascara Sagrada - Spanish explorers, suffering from constipation, were introduced to the *sacred bark* by the Native Americans. It stimulates various digestive secretions making it an excellent remedy for chronic constipation. More gentle than buckthorn, it encourages peristaltic action, relieves hemorrhoids that can be attributed to insufficient bowel movement, and is an excellent treatment for gallstones.

Cayenne - Research is underway on cayenne's active ingredient, capsaicin, which has proved to be an effective pain reliever. Its germicidal properties make it helpful with the treatment of colds and it can also act as a digestive aid. When combined with ephedra or caffeine herbs it increases metabolism thus aiding in weight loss. Boosts circulation.

Chickweed - This mild herb is used for food as well as for medicinal purposes. It is useful for bowel problems including colitis and constipation, stomach ulcers, and inflammations of the urinary tract. This very common weed also can work as an appetite depressant.

Cinnamon - Used in ancient China, India, and Egypt for diarrhea, fever, and menstrual problems, it played an important role in trade. Some experiments have demonstrated that cinnamon is very potent at stimulating insulin activity, thus aiding blood sugar. It is good for the kidneys and aids digestion by breaking down fats.

Colloidal Horsetail - Also called *shavegrass*, this fern-like plant is the sole survivor of a family that originated 200 million years ago. Rich in minerals, especially silica and selenium.

Curcumin - The coloring agent in turmeric.

Dandelion - This native of Greece is now found throughout the world. The name comes for *dens leonis*, lion's tooth, which the leaves are said to resemble. It is related to the daisy and marigold. It contains potash which is an effective diuretic, and the alkaloid, taraxacin, which is useful in the treatment of hepatitis. While diuretics deplete the body's supply of potassium, dandelion is high in potassium, making it especially useful for this purpose. In China the whole plant, including the flowers, leaves, roots, and seeds are used as a diuretic and liver stimulant. In the West the leaves and roots are used separately. It may help to reduce blood sugar, and as a bile stimulate it helps to digest fats.

Echinacea - A natural antibiotic, it is used with Chickweed to assist with weight loss.

Ephedra (Brigham Tea) - A powerful bronchial decongestant, the modern-day laboratory version is found in many over-the-counter cold remedies as *pseudoephedrine*.

Eucalyptus - A very potent herb, its leaves have antiseptic properties. Snuffing the oil will help clear sinus congestion, while mixing it with water will produce a good insect repellant.

Fennel - From the same family as carrots and parsley, it has been used since the time of the Pharaohs as a digestive aid. All parts of the plant have an anise/licorice fragrance. It has been suggested that it was used by the Puritans as an appetite suppressant, or to mask the odor of whiskey. It can be combined with herbs and used as laxatives to soothe cramps.

FoTi - strengthens the cardiovascular system, thus increasing blood flow to the heart. It is rich in flavonoids.

Garlic - has been used for at least 5000 years! It reduces blood cholesterol levels, acts as a stimulant to the immune system, and has antibiotic capabilities. The sulphur-containing compounds in garlic are what produce its very strong odor. Unfortunately, when it is deodorized, it loses many of its medicinal properties. Eating parsley or fennel after consuming garlic will help eliminate garlic breath. It is taken for bronchitis, gall bladder, and liver troubles, faintness, headaches, and skin blemishes. Its antibiotic properties have been demonstrated in some scientific studies, and, because of its use in World War II, it is referred to as Russian penicillin.

Ginger Root - Chewed by ancient Chinese sailors who discovered that it prevented sea sickness, we still use it today in the form of ginger ale and gingerbread to soothe upset stomachs. Medical tests have shown it to be more effective at treating motion sickness than Dramamine. Although it is effective in relieving morning sickness, as a smooth muscle relaxer it promotes menstruation and should therefore be used with care by pregnant women. It works well with capsicum on head and bronchial congestion.

Ginseng (Korean, Siberian, Wild American) - Known in the orient as the King of Herbs, it is considered a cure-all herb. It can be used to normalize blood pressure, reduce blood cholesterol, and prevent arteriosclerosis. It is credited with improving vision and hearing and helps to alleviate irritability. The effects of ginseng are cumulative, and consuming it for a period of time is more effective than an occasional dose.

Golden Seal - Some herbal authorities consider it to be the best general medicinal aid in the herb family. Some Native Americans (the Cherokee) used it for indigestion and local inflammations while others (the Iroquois) used it for whooping cough, fevers, and heart problems. An alkaloid, berberine, is used in a commercial eye-drop product to reduce eye irritation.

Gotu Kola - Referred to as *food for the brain*, it helps to combat stress and improve reflexes. High blood pressure, mental fatigue, and skin problems may be assuaged by Gotu Kola.

Grape Skin Extract - see Viniferous concentrate in Appendix C.

Green tea - The dried leaf of the tea plant is used to make a drink that is good for colds, congestion, asthma, and diarrhea. It is an excellent anti-oxidant and anti-allergen. Tea comes from the Greek Thea, which means goddess. When the leaf is dried and fermented it becomes black tea. Both black and green teas are sources of fluoride, which helps to prevent tooth decay.

Guarana Extract - Originating in rain forests, it is useful for extended energy.

Horseradish - A stimulant for digestion, metabolism, and kidney function, it also has an antibiotic action which is useful for urinary and respiratory infections.

Hyssop - Related to mint, hyssop is usually mixed with other herbs for best results; it helps build resistance to infections. It is useful for breast and lung conditions, coughs (from colds), poor digestion, nose and throat infections, and for intestinal mucus congestion. It inhibits herpes simplex.

Kola Nut Extract - This natural source of caffeine from Africa placates hunger and is effective in the treatment of asthma, water retention, upset stomach and diarrhea.

Licorice Root - From Greek for *sweet root*, licorice is useful in coughs, colds. Because of its very sweet taste, it is often used to mask other herbs, making them more palatable. It is used to treat stomach ulcers, and also helps to fight bacteria. In a powdered form it is put on wounds to prevent infection.

Ma-huang (Chinese Ephedra) - Used for 5,000 years in China as an anti-asthmatic. Also used for hay fever and chills. See Ephedra.

Mormon Tea - Mormon settlers were introduced to American ephedra by the Indians in Utah. It became a substitute for coffee and tea and was eventually referred to as Mormon tea. It is used for nasal and chest congestion. See Ephedra.

Peppermint - A very useful herb that is good for many remedies, it is soothing to the system, is useful in chills and colds, and will help to settle an upset stomach.

Psyllium seed - Acting as a lubricant, this gentle laxative is one of the best herbal colon cleansers.

Red Clover - Since it acts as a blood purifier, it is excellent for the entire body. Helps with acne and other skin problems and controls the appetite.

Red Korean Ginseng - One of the most expensive herbs, it can strengthen the immune system and decrease fatigue. (See ginseng.)

Rehmannia - Laxative, stops bleeding.

Reishi Mushroom - A tonic that also enhances immunity, it has been effective in relieving the side effects of chemotherapy. Regulates blood sugar. Anti-oxidant.

Sarsaparilla - Increases the metabolic rate and balances hormones. Since it contains a chemical called *saponins,* which causes a diuretic action, it is useful in the treatment of high blood pressure and congestive heart disease. It was discovered by Spanish explorers in the Caribbean who gave it the name *zaraz* (prickly), *parra* (vine), *illa* (small). Cowboys in the old west asked for sarsaparilla mistakenly believing that it was a treatment for syphilis. An extract has proved beneficial for psoriasis.

Senna leaves - increase intestinal peristalsis, thus making it a stimulating laxative. A bad-tasting herb often combined with ginger or fennel to prevent bowel cramps, it is an ingredient in many over-the-counter laxatives.

Siberian Ginseng - see Ginseng

Turmeric (tumeric) - From Asia, this plant is related to ginger. The root is the useful part of the plant and was used as a dye for fabric and to give a yellow tint to rice and other foods.

Uva Ursi (bear berry) - strengthens the urinary system, making is useful for bladder and kidney infections and stones. The ancient Asians, Europeans, and Native Americans were all aware of the diuretic properties of this bitter herb, which is also good for female disorders. It contains allantoin, which promotes the growth of healthy new cells and is the active ingredient in over-the-counter creams for herpes (oral) and vaginal infections.

Uncaria Tomentosa (Cat's Claw) - from the Peruvian Amazon, has been used by natives for hundreds of years to treat immune and digestive system problems. Research on this plant is now being done at a number of locations around the world and indicates that cat's claw may be useful in the treatment of cancer, arthritis, bursitis, genital herpes, allergies, ulcers, system candidiasis, PMS, and various bowel disorders. One source reports that it alleviated a 20-year old chronic urinary track problem.

White Willow - see Willow

Willow - A natural *aspirin* that is mild on the stomach, it is used for fever and chills. White willow bark was used in ancient Egypt for minor aches, pains, and fever. It is useful for stomach troubles, especially heartburn.

Yerba Mate - Rich in vitamins, this herb from South America contains no caffeine but alleviates fatigue and helps to protect the body from the effects of stress. It aids allergy symptoms by opening respiratory passages.

Yerba Santa - Although mild, this is a useful decongestant for all forms of bronchial congestion. It stimulates digestive secretions, including the salivary glands.

AMINO ACIDS

Essential Amino Acids:

Branch Chain Aminos - called the stress amino acids, they are needed for energy, hemoglobin, and to stabilize blood sugar.

Histidine - is essential in infants but only semi-essential in adults. It helps form histamine, important to immune system, production of blood cells, and aids copper transport through joints.

Lysine - helps rebuild muscle and repairs damaged tissue, assists in calcium absorption for bone growth, collagen formation, hormones and enzymes.

Methionine - a source of organic sulphur for healthy liver, lymph, and immune system, it supports healthy skin and nails and prevents hair loss.

Phenylalanine - works with B-6 as an anti-depressant and mood elevator, aids learning and memory, and stimulates the thyroid.

Threonine - an immune stimulant and thymus enhancer, this amino acid is necessary for collagen formation.

Tryptophan - involved in mood and metabolism regulation.

Tyrosine - helps build adrenalin and thyroid hormones, is a source of quick energy; converts to L-Dopa amino acid, which improves brain function.

Non-essential Or Semi-essential Amino Acids:

Arginine - growth hormone stimulant, it increases muscle tone while decreasing fat, and promotes wound healing.

Carnitine - stimulates enzymes to help regulate metabolism of fat, provides energy to heart muscle, increases oxidation of fat for weight loss and energy.

Ornithine - along with arginine and carnitine it helps to metabolize excess fat; aids pituitary gland in production of growth hormone for muscle development; strengthens immune system and fights free radicals.

OTHER TREASURES

"For there exist in our possession hidden treasures in the field, wheat and barley and oil and honey."

- Jeremiah 41:8

Acidophilus is a "friendly" bacteria that aids digestion and assimilation of nutrients. Some research suggests that it may also prevent colon cancer.

Aloe extract- aloe may look like some cacti, but actually it is a member of the lilacea family which includes lilies and onions. The gel from the cut leaf of the aloe is excellent on burns and other wounds. The leaves have a laxative effect and stimulate bile flow and digestion.

Aloe Vera is a mucopolysaccharide, an essential factor for cellular resistance to viruses and pathogenic bacteria. Mucopolysaccharides provide needed lubrication of joints and they aid the body in absorbing water, minerals, and nutrients in the intestinal track. Since they are produced by the body only through puberty, adults must obtain them from other sources.

Bee Pollen is said to contain every substance needed to maintain life. Bees collect the pollen of male seed flowers, mix it with a secretion, and form it into granules. A blood building and rejuvenating substance, it aids respiratory problems, chronic colitis, constipation, diarrhea, nervous and endocrine system complaints, and boosts healing.

Only unsprayed pollen should be used for therapeutic purposes. Start with small doses to ascertain that the individual is not allergic to the bee pollen.

Bentonite is a clay substance that absorbs toxins and bacteria. It is used for intestinal cleaning.

Biotin, the crystalline vitamin in yeast, is one of the B vitamins. It is needed for healthy hair and skin. It aids in cell growth and improves glucose tolerance in diabetics.

Bromelin, an enzyme found in pineapple, aids digestion by breaking down fat. It stimulates metabolism.

Collagen is the protein in the cartilage and other connective tissues of animals. It is rich in proline, a non-essential amino acid.

Chromium is essential, even in trace amounts, for proper glucose regulation. It enhances the use of insulin, so it is effective in controlling cravings for sugar. It also helps the body burn fat while increasing lean muscle formation, making it a key nutrient for dieters.

Enzymes are required for everything the body does -- seeing, thinking, smelling, breathing, tasting, talking, playing and walking, to name just a few. Life without enzymes is not possible because they are in every living thing.

Most enzymes are manufactured in the body by the proteins and there are two types of these: metabolic and digestive. Metabolic enzymes run the body and make repairs. Digestive enzymes help process carbohydrates and fat and turn them into fuel the body can use.

A third type of enzyme is found in raw foods. They start food digestion and help the body's own digestive enzymes so they don't have to work so hard. Enzymes, which are really sophisticated proteins, won't work by themselves. They need help from vitamins or minerals to get their jobs done.

Hesperidium is in the fruit of a citrus plant. Suggested daily dose is 100 mg.

Luecocyanadins (grape seed extract) raises HDL (the good) cholesterol.

Oat bran is produced from the coarse husks of the grain's seed. A soluble fiber in oat bran, beta glucans, interferes with the production and absorption of cholesterol. Consumption of oat bran will help lower LDL, increase HDL, and provide needed fiber for the intestinal track.

Papain - An enzyme from papaya trees, it breaks down protein so that it can be digested. For this reason it is eaten after meals to enhance digestion. The juice has been used to dissolve corns, warts, and pimples. It will relieve a sour stomach.

Pectin - A gelatinous substance found in fruit, it lowers LDL and increases HDL cholesterol. In one study, rats fed pectin had a 50% drop in colon cancer. Apple pectin adds bulk to the stool, thus relieving both diarrhea and constipation. It helps control blood sugar levels and binds with some cancer-causing compounds in the colon, thus speeding their elimination from the body.

Royal Jelly is a substance secreted from glands located on the heads of honeybee workers. It is fed to the future queen bees. A natural anti-biotic, it stimulates the immune system, and as one of the richest sources of pantothenic acid, it will combat stress and fatigue, aid digestion, and produce healthy skin and hair.

Viniferous concentrate (grape skin extract) is derived from the European grape cultivated in the western United States.

DIETS

The amounts of carbohydrates, proteins and fat
recommended in some popular diets today:

Diet	Protein	Carbs	Fat
HCF	23.5	65.5	11
Pritikin	14	74	12
Gluten	12	58	30
Lactose Free	15	59	26
Hyper.Child	16	58	26
Low Trigly.	17	65	18
Immune Enh.	20	50	30
Ornish	15	75	10
McDougall	10	85	5
Mean:	15.8	65.5	18.7

BIBLIOGRAPHY

FOR APPENDIX A – HERBS:

Herbs for All Seasons, Sally Freeman,
The Penguin Group, New York, 1991.

Today's Herbal Health, 3rd Edition, Louise Tenney, M.H.
Woodland Books, Provo, UT 1992.

Food - Your Miracle Medicine, Jean Carper,
Harper Collins Publishers, Inc., New York 1993.

*The Healing Herbs - The Ultimate Guide to the Curative
Power of Nature's Medicines*, Michael Castleman,
Rodale Books, Emmaus, PA, 1991.

Healthy Healing, Linda Rector-Page
Healthy Healing Publications, 1992.

The Complete Book of Herbs and Spices, Claire
Loewenfeld and Philippa Back
G.P. Putnam's Sons, New York 1974

Miracle Medicine Herbs, Richard Melvin Lucas,
Parker Publishing Company, West Nyack, NY 1991

The Complete Medicinal Herbal, Penelope Ody,
Dorling Kindersely, Inc., New York, 1993

A Useful Guide to Herbal Health Care, Health Center for
Better Living, Inc., Naples, FL

FOR CHAPTERS

BARICE, E. Joan, MD with Kathleen Jonck, *The Palm Beach Long-Life Diet.* New York: Simon & Shuster, 1988.

BATMANGHELIDJ, F., MD, *Your Body's Many Cries for Water.* Falls Church, VA: Global Health Solutions, Inc., 1992.

BENDER, Arnold E., PhD, *Health or Hoax.* Buffalo, New York: Prometheus Books, 1986.

BERGER, Stuart M., MD, Dr. Berger's Immune Power Diet. New York: New American Library, 1985.

BISHOP, Jerry E., "Evidence of Dependence on Caffeine Found in Some Participants in Study." *The Wall Street Journal,* October 5, 1944.

BLAND, Dr. Jeffrey, *Nutraerobics.* New York: Harper & Row Publishers, Inc. 1983.

BRECHER, Harold and Arlene, *Forty Something Forever – A Consumer's Guide to Chelation Therapy.* Herndon, VA: Healthsavers Press, September 1994.

BRICKLIN, Mark, *The Practical Encyclopedia of Natural Healing.* Emmaus, PA: Rodale Press, 1983.

BROOKS, R.T., *Ask the Bible.* New York: Gramercy Publishing Company, 1989.

BROWNLEE, Shannon, "The Cellular Battlefield." *U.S. News & World Report,* March 28, 1994.

CARTER, James P., MD, Dr. P.H., *Racketeering In Medicine: The Suppression of Alternatives.* Norfolk, VA: Hampton Roads Publishing Company, Inc., 1992.

COCHRAN, Patrick E., "Beef Up Your Diet with the Master Key to Health." *Senior Highlights,* September 1994.

COUSENS, Gabriel, MD, *Spiritual Nutrition and the Rainbow Diet.* Boulder, CO: Cassandra Press, 1986.

DIAMOND, Harvey and Marilyn, *Fit for Life II: Living Health.* New York: Warner Books, 1987.

DRACKER, Pune, "Heal Spot, Heal." *ASPCA Animal Watch,* Fall 1994.

DUFTY, William, *Sugar Blues.* New York: Warner Books, 1975.

FITZGERALD, Frances E., "Understanding Homeopathy." *Health Counselor,* Vol. 5, No. 2.

FLEXNER, Abraham, *Abraham Flexner, An Autobiography.* New York: Simon & Shuster, Inc., 1960.

FRISBY, Bill, ND, D.Sc, *God's HMO.* Dunwoody, GA: Metabiotics, 1990.

GOOCH, Sandy, *If You Love Me Don't Feed Me Junk.* Reston, VA: Reston Publishing Company, Inc., 1988.

HAAS, Dr. Robert, *Eat to Win, The Sports Nutrition Bible.* New York: Rawson Associates, 1983.

HARDIE, Ann, "Prescribed drugs make one in four elderly people ill." Atlanta, GA: *The Atlanta Constitution,* July 27, 1994.

IDONE, Christopher, *Glorious American Food.* New York: Random House, 1985.

JAMPOLSKY, Gerald G., MD and Diane V. Cirincione, *Love is the Answer.* New York: Bantam Books, 1990.

LANDE, Nathaniel, *Self Health.* New York: Holt, Rinehart and Winston, 1980.

LEHMAN, Phyllis, "More Than You Ever Thought You Would Know About Food Additives...Part II and Part III." *FDA Consumer,* U.S. Department of Health, Education and Welfare, 1979.

LIEBERMAN, Shari and BRUNING, Nancy, *The Real Vitamin & Mineral Book.* Garden City Park, NY: Avery Publishing Group, Inc., 1990.

McDOUGALL, John A., MD, and Mary A., *The McDougall Plan.* Clinton, NJ: New Win Publishing Co., Inc., 1983.

MILLER, Leslie, "Getting iron out of kids' reach," *USA Today,* October 6, 1994.

MILLER, Leslie, "Guides for treating ailments naturally," *USA Today,* September 6, 1994.

MORTER, Dr. M. Ted, Jr., *Your Health, Your Choice.* Hollywood FL: Fell Publishers, Inc., 1990.

MOWREY, Daniel B., PhD, *Next Generation Herbal Medicine.* New Canaan, CT: Keats Publishing, Inc., 1990.

NEAG, Ray, "Catheter Helps Prevent Sepsis in Bloodstream." New York: *The Wall Street Journal,* September 27, 1994.

NEWMAN, Dr. Laura, *Make Your Juicer Your Drugstore.* New York: Benedict Lust Publications, 1978.

ORNISH, Dean, MD, *Eat More, Weigh Less.* New York: Harper Collins Publishers, Inc., 1993.

PECK, M. Scott, MD, *The Road Less Traveled.* New York: Simon & Shuster, 1978.

PRITIKIN, Nathan, *Diet for Runners.* New York: Simon & Shuster, 1985.

READER'S DIGEST, *ABC's of the Human Mind.* Pleasantville, NY: The Reader's Digest Association, Inc., 1990.

READER'S DIGEST, *How in the World.* Pleasantville, NY: The Reader's Digest Association, Inc., 1990.

RECTOR-PAGE, Linda, ND, PhD, *Healthy Healing.* Healthy Healing Publications, Inc., 1992.

REUBEN, David, MD, *Everything You Always Wanted to Know about Nutrition.* New York: Simon & Shuster, 1978.

RITTER, Lee, *Aloe Vera, A Mission Discovered.* Northglen, CO: Lee Ritter, 1993.

ROBBINS, John, *Diet for a New America.* Walpole, NH: Stillpoint Publishing, 1987.

U.S. DEPARTMENT OF HEALTH AND HUMAN SERVICES, *The Surgeon General's Report on Nutrition and Health.* New York: Warner Books, Inc., May 1989.

RONA, Zoltan P., MD, *The Joy of Health.* St. Paul, MN: Llewellyn Publications, Inc., 1994.

SAMUELS, Mike, MD, and Nancy Samuels, *The Well Adult.* New York: Summit Books, 1988.

SEABROOK, Charles, "1 in 3 Americans weighs too much." Atlanta, GA: *The Atlanta Constitution,* July 20, 1994.

SHAHEEN, Carol Ann, "Minerals Men Need." *Men's Health,*
September, 1994.

SHELDON, Margen, MD, and the Editors of "University of
California at Berkley Wellness Letter." *The Wellness Encyclopedia
of Food and Nutrition.* New York: Rubus, 1992.

SIMONE, Charles B., MD, *Cancer & Nutrition.* Garden City Park,
NY: Avery Publishing Group, 1992.

Sodium, Think About It, United States Department of Agriculture and
United States Department of Health and Human Services: 1982.

Sulfite Sensitivity & Eating Out, National Restaurant Association and
the Food Allergy Committee of the American College of Allergists.

Surviving the 90's with Good Health, Healthexcel, Inc.,
Washington, DC, 1989.

The Surgeon General's Report on Nutrition and Health, U.S.
Department of Health and Human Resources. New York: Warner
Books, Inc., 1989.

The Tufts University Guide to Total Nutrition. New York: Harper &
Row Publishers, 1990.

University of California at Berkley Wellness Letter, Vol. II, Issue I,
October 1994.

INDEX

Endnotes

1 Newman, Dr. Laura., *Make Your Juicer Your Drug Store*, Benedict Lust Publications, July 1978 edition, p. 20.

2 Flexner, Abraham, *Abraham Flexner An Autobiography*. New York: Simon & Shuster, Inc. 1960. p. 77.

3 Flexner, p. 87.

4 Diamond, Harvey & Marilyn, *Fit for Life II: Living Health*. New York, NY: Warner Books, 1987. p. 16.

5 Diamond, p. 16.

6 *Wall Street Journal*, October 5, 1994, p. B1.

7 *USA Today*, July 27, 1994, p. 1.

8 Hardie, Ann, "Prescribed drugs make one in four elderly people ill" *The Atlanta Constitution*, July 27, 1994. p. 1.

9 Neag, Ray, "Catheter Helps Prevent Sepsis in Bloodstream," *The Wall Street Journal*, September 27, 1994.

10 Seabrook, Charles, "1 in 3 Americans weighs too much," *The Atlanta Journal/Atlanta Constitution*, July 20, 1994. p. B1.
11 Newman, p. 21.

12 Dufty, William, *Sugar Blues*. New York, NY: Warner Books, 1975. p. 69.

13 Morter, Dr. M. Ted, Jr., *Your Health Your Choice*. Hollywood, FL: Fell Publishers, Inc. 1990, p. 115.

14 Morter, xxiv
15 Newman, p. 7.

16 Simone, Charles, B., M.D., *Cancer & Nutrition*. Garden City Park, NY: Avery Publishing Groups, Inc., 1992. p. 115.

17 Simone, p. 116.

18 Simone, p. 116.

19 Robbins, John, *Diet for a New America*. Walpole, NH: Stillpoint International, Inc., 1987. p. 164.

20 Morter, p. 106.

21 Rector-Page, Linda, N.D., Ph.D., *Healthy Healing*, p. 63

22 Rector-Page, p. 63.

23 Simone, p. 193.

24 Diamond, p. 103.

25 Rona, Zoltan P., M.D., M.Sc., *The Joy of Health*. St. Paul, MN: Llewellyn Publications, 1994. p. 50.

26 Simone, p. 193.

27 Batmanghelidj, F., M.D., *Your Body's Many Cries for Water*, Global Health Solutions, Inc., 1992, p. 123.

28 Batmanghelidj, p. 123.

29 Batmanghelidj, p. 10.

30 Diamond, p. 29.

31 Morter, p. 72.

32 Simone, p. 38.

33 Lande, Nathaniel, *Self Health*. New York: Holt, Rinehart and Winston, 1980, p. 37.

34 Morter, p. 117.

35 McDougall, John A., M.D. and Mary A., *The McDougall Plan*. New Win Publishing, Inc., Clinton, NJ: 1983. p. 96.

36 McDougall. p. 97.

37 Cochran, Patrick E., "Beef Up Your Diet with the Master Key to Health," *Senior Highlights*, September 1994, pp. 7, 8.

38 Morter, p. 121.

39 Cousens, Gabriel, M.D., *Spiritual Nutrition and the Rainbow Diet*. Boulder, CO: Cassandra Press, 1986, p. 131.

40 Lieberman, Shari and Bruning, Nancy, *The Real Vitamin & Mineral Book*. Garden City Park, New York: Avery Publishing Group, Inc. 1990, p. xii.

41 Lande, Nathaniel, *Self Health*. New York: Holt, Rinehart and Winston, 1980. p. 44.

42 Lande, p. 32

43 Lande, p. 42.

44 Shaheen, Carol Ann, "Minerals Men Need." *Men's Health*, September 1994. p. 50.

45 Miller, Leslie, "Getting iron out of kids' reach," *USA Today*, October 6, 1994, p. D1.

46 Rector-Page, p. 30.

47 Rector-Page, p. 23.

48 Rector-Page, p. 30.

49 Reader's Digest, *How In The World*. Pleasantville, NY: The Reader's Digest Association, Inc., 1990. p. 366.

50 Brownlee, Shannon, "The cellular battlefield," *U.S. News & World Report*, March 28, 1994, p. 66.

51 Lande, p. 44.

52 Reader's Digest, *ABC's of the Human Mind.* Pleasantville, New York: The Reader's Digest Association, Inc. 1990. p. 134.

53 Lande, p. 103.
54 *University of California at Berkeley Wellness Letter*, Vol. 11, Issue 1, October 1994. pp. 3.

55 Lande, p. 108.

56 Simone, p. 204.

57 Simone, p. 204.

58 Goodwin, Jan, "Is it Voo-Doo?" New Woman, October 1994, p. 111.
59 Goodwin, Jan, p. 113
60 *USA Today*, July 27, 1994. p. 1.

61 http://www.prlog.org/11905119-drugs-with-the-most-frequent-reports-of-adverse-reactions.html

62 Rona, p. 9.
63 FitzGerald, Frances E., "Understanding Homeopathy," *Health Counselor*, Vol. 5, No. 2, pp. 23, 24.

64 FitzGerald, p. 24.

65 Dracker, Pune, "Heal Spot, Heal." *ASPCA Animal Watch*, Fall 1994, p. 20.

66 Ritter, Leo, *Aloe Vera, A Mission Discovered.* Northglen, CO: Lee Ritter, 1993. p. 17.

67 Miller, Leslie, *USA Today*, "Guides for treating ailments naturally." September 6, 1994, p. 6D.

68 http://www.usatoday.com/news/health/2007-03-13-cancer-boom_N.htm
69 Simone, p. 3.

70 Rona, p. 11.

71 Brownlee, Shannon, "The cellular battlefield," *U.S. News & World Report*, March 28, 1994. p. 66.

72 http://www.sharecare.com/question/sugar-consume-every-year

73 http://www.stopsmokingbible.com/how-many-people-in-america-smoke-cigarettes

74 http://www.learn-about-alcoholism.com/statistics-on-alcoholics.html

75 Bishop, Jerry E., "Evidence of Dependence on Caffeine Found in Some Participants in Study" *The Wall Street Journal*, October 5, 1994, p. B6.

76 Dufty, William, *Sugar Blues*. New York, NY: Warner Books, 1975. p. 28.

77 Dufty, p. 31.

78 Dufty, p. 30.

78 Rona, p. 113.

79 Reader's Digest, *ABC's of the Human Mind*, The Reader's Digest Association, Pleasantville, New York, 1990. p. 83.

80 Rona, p. 47.

81 *Los Angeles Times*, September 30, 1986.

83 Mindell, Dr. Earl. What You Should Know about Beautiful Hair, Skin and Nails. Keats Publishing, Inc., New Canaan, Ct., 1996. p. 7.
84 Ibid, p. 8.

85 Rector-Page, Linda G., N.D., Ph.D.. Ibid. p. 226.

86 Tenney, Louise, M.H. Today's Herbal Health, Third Edition. Woodland Books, Provo, UT. 1992. p. 267.

87 Tenney, Louise, M.H. Today's Herbal Health, Third Edition. Woodland Books, Provo, UT. 1992. p. 267.

88 Mindell, Ibid. p. 65.

89 Jones, Susan Smith, Ph.D. "Beauty: Make it Skin Deep," Let's Live, June 1996. p. 36.

90 Goldway, Elliot M., Ph.D. The Joy of Life. Octopus Books Ltd., 1978.

91 Rector-Page, Linda G., N.D., Ph.D.. Ibid. p. 226.

92 Mindell, Dr. Earl. Ibid. p. 62.

93 http://latimesblogs.latimes.com/alltherage/2012/02/brazilian-blowout-to-carry-warning-labels.html

94 http://going-well.com/2010/02/03/14-toxic-chemicals-to-avoid-in-skin-care-and-hair-care-products-including-organic/